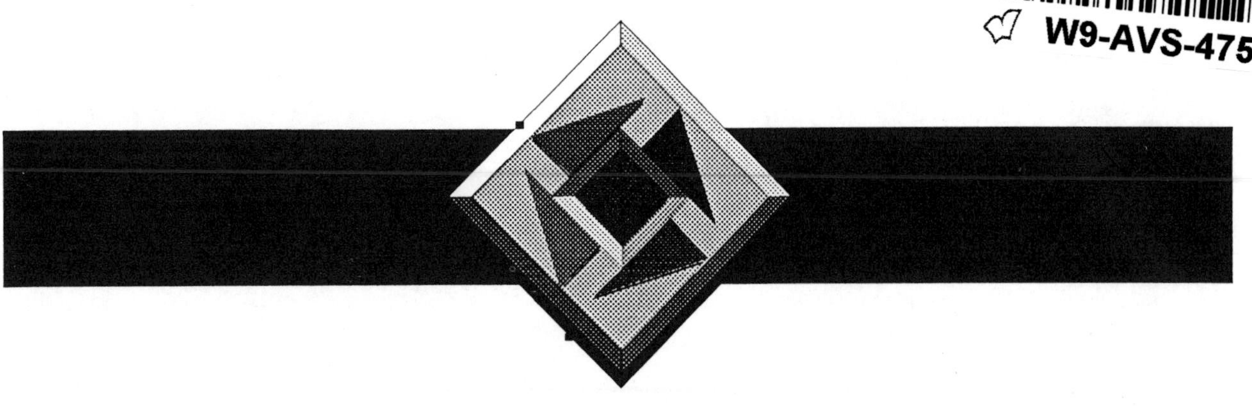

INSTRUCTORS MANUAL

by Ray A.Petersen and Norene C. Petersen
Brigham Young University

FOR

Lifetime Physical Fitness and Wellness

A Personalized Program

FOURTH EDITION

Werner W. K. Hoeger
Bosie State University

Sharon A. Hoeger

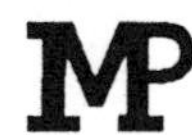

MORTON PUBLISHING COMPANY
925 W. Kenyon, Unit 12
Englewood, Colorado 80110

Printed in the United States of America
10 9 8 7 6 5 4 3 2 1
ISBN: 0–89582–292–X

Preface

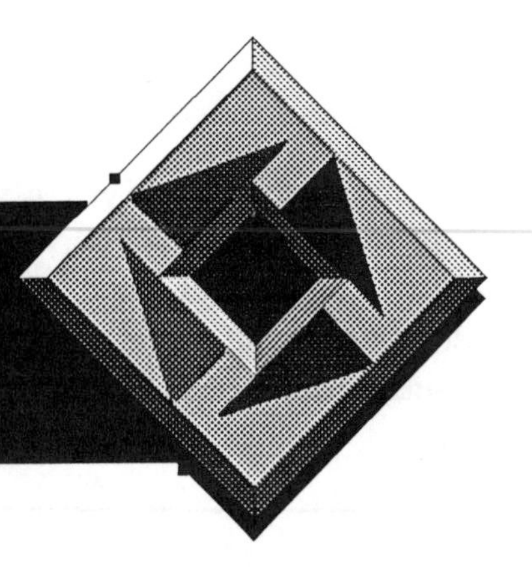

This instructor's manual was prepared to accompany the textbook, *Lifetime Physical Fitness and Wellness: A personalized Program*, written by and Werner W. K. Hoeger and Sharon A. Hoeger published by Morton Publishing Company. Each of the chapters in this manual contain the following features.

Student Objectives. The instructors attention is directed to the student objectives listed in the text at the begining of each chapter. To conserve space they are not repeated in this manual. However, they give both the student and the instructor a view of what the student is expected to be able to know and do when the chapter is completed.

Expanded Chapter Outline. This is a very comprehensive outline of the material covered in the chapter. An instructor could use it as lecture notes, and perhaps highlight the parts of the outline of particular significance.

Instructor Activities. A few possible teaching activities are suggested for each chapter. Many of these activities center around the use of an overhead projector.

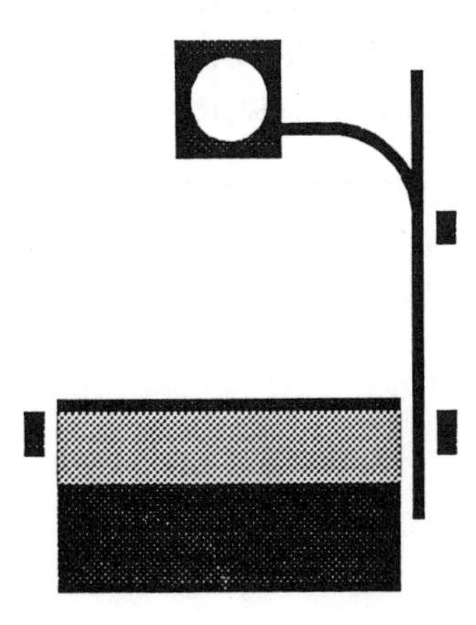

The Instructor Activities also refer to transparency masters in this manual. These were prepared by Ray A. Petersen. In some cases clip art from WordPerfect Corporation and New Vision Technologies Inc. were used. An instructor can use a copy machine and clear or color plastic or acetate sheets to make copies that can be used with an overhead projector.

SUPPLEMENTS

The following ancillaries are provided free of charge to all qualified *Lifetime Physical Fitness & Wellness* adopters:

- The Fitness & Wellness Profile Plus includes a *Fitness and Wellness Profile, a Personalized Cardiovascular Exercise Prescription*, a *Nutrient Analysis*, and a weekly and monthly *Exercise Log*. This software package helps provide a more meaningful experience to all participants and greatly decreases the workload of course instructors.

  A new feature of the fourth edition is the *Nutrient Analysis Data Base Enhancer* software. This software allows instructors to add food items to the already existing data base available with the book.

- A **video** containing a detailed explanation of many of the fitness assessment test items used in the book. Instructors can use this video to help familiarize themselves with the proper test protocols for each fitness test. This audio-visual aid contains the following test items: 1.5-Mile Run Test, Step Test, Astrand-Ryhming Test, Muscular Strength and Endurance Test, Muscular Endurance Test, Strength-to-Body Weight Ratio Test, Modified Sit-and-Reach Test, Body Rotation Test, Shoulder Rotation Test, Skinfold Thickness Test, and Girth Measurements Test.

- The Physical Fitness and Wellness Computerized Testbank with the following options: (a) over 800 multiple choice questions, (b) capability to add/or edit test questions, (c) previously generated tests can be recalled — creating new exam versions because multiple choice answers can be rotated with each new test generated, and (d) capability to generate tests using a LaserJet printer.

- Sixty-four color **overhead transparency acetates** of the book's most important illustrations and figures to facilitate class instruction and help explain key fitness and wellness concepts.

Contents

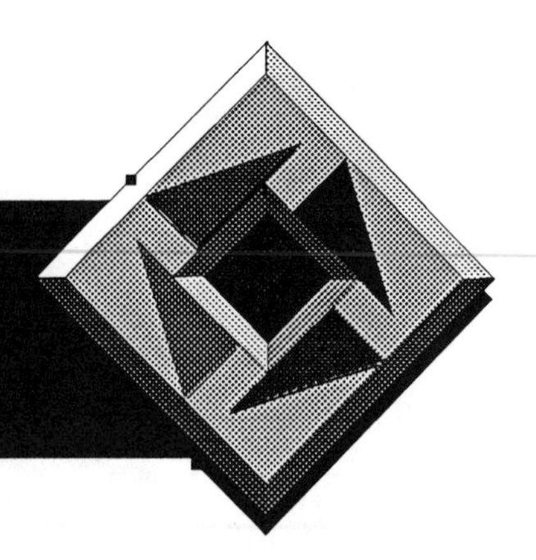

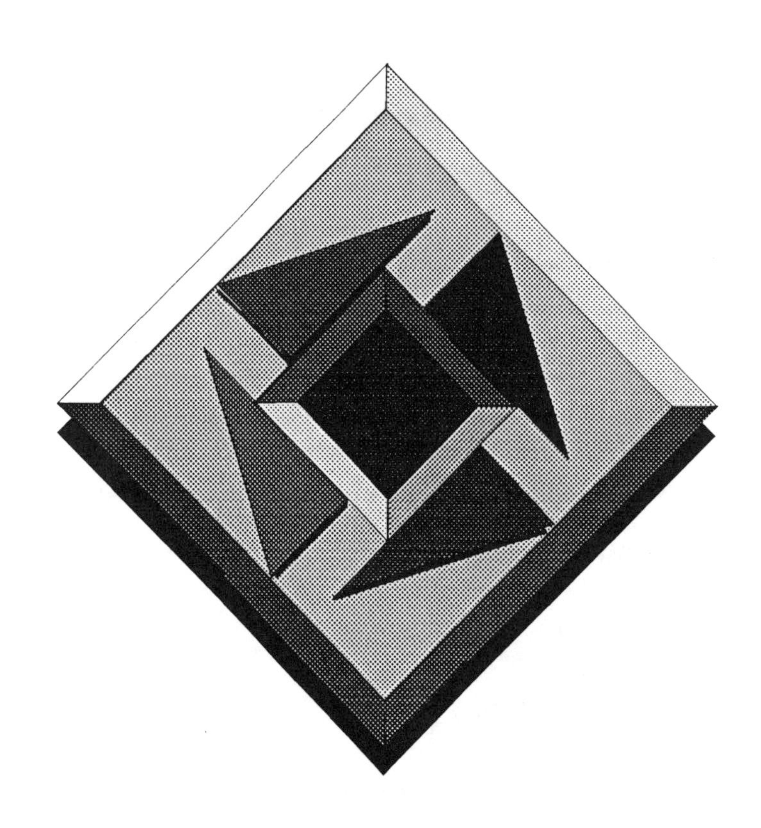

Introduction to Lifetime Physical Fitness and Wellness

1

Expanded Chapter Outline

I. CHANGING LIFESTYLES

A. The most common health problems in the U.S. have changed since the beginning of the 20th century.

1. In 1900 infection was the leading cause of disease.
2. Recent progress in medicine has largely eliminated such diseases.
3. However, there has been an increase in chronic diseases.
4. As the incidence of chronic diseases increased, prevention emerged as the best medicine.

B. Since American people started to enjoy the "good life," four factors have negatively affected human health:

1. Sedentary lifestyle
    a. Movement and physical activity are basic to good health.
    b. Physical inactivity is a serious threat to our health.
    c. Over 250,000 deaths yearly are the result from the lack of regular physical activity.
2. Poor nutrition
3. Stress
4. Environment

C. As people realized that good health is largely self-controlled, a fitness and wellness trend began to develop.

1. Premature death and illness in the United States could be prevented by adhering to positive lifestyle habits.
2. Participating in a wellness program improves quality of life.
    a. improving physical fitness

b. watching body weight
c. avoiding high blood pressure
d. controlling stress
e. avoiding tobacco and too much alcohol
f. avoiding too many fatty foods

II. WELLNESS

A. The wellness concept developed in the 1980s.

1. Good health is no longer is viewed as simply the absence of illness.
2. Scientists have learned that lifestyle factors affect wellness.
3. Wellness is defined as the constant and deliberate effort to stay healthy and achieve the highest potential for well-being.
4. Wellness requires the implementation of positive programs to change behavior.
5. To enjoy wellness, a person needs to practice behaviors that will lead to positive outcomes in five dimensions of wellness:
    a. physical
    b. emotional
    c. intellectual
    d. social
    e. spiritual
6. These dimensions are interrelated; one frequently affects the others.
7. Wellness incorporates components such as:
    a. fitness
    b. proper nutrition
    c. stress management
    d. disease prevention
    e. social support
    f. self-worth nurturance (sense of being needed)
    g. spirituality
    h. smoking cessation
    i. personal safety
    j. substance control
    k. regular physical examinations
    l. health education
    m. environmental support

III. PHYSICAL FITNESS

A. Comprehensive definition of physical fitness:

1. The general capacity to adapt and respond favorably to physical effort (AMA).
2. Individuals are physically fit when they can:
    a. meet the ordinary as well as the unusual demands of daily life
    b. safely and effectively without being overly fatigued

c. and still have energy left for leisure and recreational activities

B. A battery of tests, not a single test, is necessary to determine an individual'soverall level of fitness.

C. The health-related fitness components (important in prevention) are:
1. cardiovascular (aerobic) endurance
2. muscular strength and endurance
3. muscular flexibility
4. body composition

D. Motor skill-related fitness (important in athletics) includes:
1. agility
2. balance
3. coordination
4. power
5. reaction time
6. speed

IV. THE WELLNESS APPROACH

A. A decrease in cardiovascular mortality rates is credited to higher levels of wellness.
1. Several studies have shown an inverse relationship between exercise and premature cardiovascular mortality rates.
2. Healthy lifestyle habits include abstaining from tobacco, alcohol, caffeine, and drugs.

B. Adhering to a well-balanced diet:
- a. based on grains
- b. fruits and vegetables
- c. moderate consumption of poultry and red meat

V. HEALTH FITNESS VERSUS PHYSICAL FITNESS STANDARDS

A. A health fitness standard:
1. Moderate aerobic exercise provides significant health benefits
   - a. a reduction in blood lipids
   - b. lower blood pressure
   - c. less risk for diabetes
   - d. weight loss
   - e. stress release
   - f. lower risk for disease and premature mortality
2. Examples of moderate physical activity for cardiovascular endurance:

a. A 2-mile walk in less than 30 minutes, five to six times per week, seems to be sufficient to achieve the health-fitness standard.
b. Cardiovascular endurance is measured in terms of the maximal amount of oxygen the body is able to utilize per minute of physical activity.

B. Physical-Fitness Standards

1. Physical fitness standards require more vigorous exercise.
2. Those with "good" physical fitness should be able to do moderate to vigorous physical activity without undue fatigue.
3. They should be able to maintain this capability throughout life.
   a. Older people should be able to do similar activities to those they did in their youth, though not with the same intensity.
   b. A person does not have to be an elite athlete, he or she should be above the "average fitness" level of the American people.

VI. LEADING HEALTH PROBLEMS IN THE UNITED STATES

A. The prominent causes of death in the U. S. are lifestyle-related.

1. Cardiovascular disease and cancer are the first and second leading causes of death in this country.
   a. They account for 70% of all deaths in this country.
   b. Nearly 80% of these deaths could be prevented through a healthy lifestyle.
2. The third leading cause of death, chronic and obstructive pulmonary disease, is related largely to tobacco use.
3. Accidents are the fourth leading cause of death.
   a. Many accidents are preventable.
   b. They are often related to drug abuse.
   c. They are often related to not wearing seat belts.

B. Based on current figures:

1. A tenth of all disease is attributed to improper health care.
2. A fifth is attributed to the environment.
3. About 16% is related to genetic factors.
4. More than half of disease is lifestyle-related.
5. Thus, the individual controls 84% of disease and quality of life.

C. Cardiovascular Disease

1. The most prevalent degenerative diseases in the United States are those of the cardiovascular system.
2. Almost half of all deaths in this country are attributed to heart and blood vessel disease.
3. By 1990, AHA estimates more than 70 million Americans were afflicted with diseases of the cardiovascular system.

a. 63.6 million with hypertension
b. 6.2 million with coronary heart disease

4. The estimated cost of this disease exceeded $117 billion including lost industrial productivity.
5. About a million and a half people have heart attacks each year and a third of those people die as a consequence.
   a. About half the time the first symptom of coronary heart disease is the heart attack itself.
   b. And 40% of those who have a first heart attack die within the first 24 hours.
   c. About half of the people who die are men in their most productive years, between ages 40 and 65.

D. Cancer

1. The second leading cause of death in the United States is cancer.
2. The mortality rate for cancer has increased steadily.
3. Cancer is the number-one health fear of the American people.
4. Approximately 23% of all deaths in the United States is from cancer.
5. Almost 526,000 people died from this disease in 1993.
6. The 1990 medical costs for cancer were estimated at $104 billion.

E. Chronic Obstructive Pulmonary Disease

1. Chronic obstructive pulmonary disease (COPD) refers to diseases that limit air flow.
2. It includes chronic bronchitis, emphysema, and conditions such as asthma.
3. The incidence of COPD increases proportionately with cigarette smoking and exposure to certain types of industrial pollution.

F. Accidents

1. Accidents are the fourth leading cause of death in the U. S.
2. Accident prevention and personal safety are also a part of a health enhancement program.
3. Most accidents do not just happen, they are caused.
   a. Some accidents such as earthquakes, tornadoes, and airplane crashes are beyond our control.
   b. Most accidents are the result of poor judgment and confused mental states.
4. Alcohol abuse is the number-one cause of all accidents.

VII. BENEFITS OF A COMPREHENSIVE WELLNESS PROGRAM

A. Health Benefits:

1. Improves personal appearance and self-esteem.
2. Active people generally live longer.
3. Physically fit individuals enjoy a better quality of life:
   a. They live life to its fullest.

b. They have fewer health problems.

B. Economic Benefits:

1. As the need for physical exertion steadily decreased during the last century, the nation's health-care expenditures increased dramatically.
2. Health-care costs in the United States rose from $12 billion in 1950 to approximately $738 billion in 1992.
3. If the rate of escalation continues, health-care expenditures will reach $1.6 trillion by the year 2002.
4. In 1992 the cost of personal health care represented more than 12% of the gross national product (GNP).
5. It is projected to reach about 18% by the year 2002 and 37% by 2030.
6. Evidence now links participation in fitness and wellness programs to:
    a. better health.
    b. lower medical costs.
    c. higher job productivity.
7. Approximately one-half of the health-care expenditures in the United States are being absorbed by American business and industry.
    a. Many organizations realize that keeping employees healthy costs less than treating them once they are sick.
    b. Containing the costs of health care through fitness and wellness programs has become a major issue for many organizations.
    c. Some organizations offer wellness programs simply because they are concerned for the physical well-being of employees.
    d. Wellness programs help individuals feel better about themselves and improve their quality of life.
    e. Some executives believe that an on-site health promotion program is the best fringe benefit they can offer.

VIII. THE WELLNESS CHALLENGE FOR THE FUTURE

A. A better and healthier life is something every person should strive for.

B. Our challenge is to teach people how to take control of their personal health habits and adhere to a positive lifestyle.

C. Improving the quality of life is a matter of personal choice.

D. Research indicates that to significantlyimprove health and extend life, a person should:

1. Participate in a lifetime exercise program.
2. Not smoke cigarettes or use smokeless tobacco products.
3. Eat right.
4. Maintain recommended body weight.
5. Get enough rest. Sleep 7 to 8 hours each night.

6. Lower stress levels as needed.
7. Be wary of alcohol.
8. Surround yourself with healthy friendships.
9. Be informed about the environment.
10. Take personal safety measures.

E. **Most Americans now see a need for a personal wellness program but many are not participating properly.**
   1. Some are not participating because they are unaware of the basic principles for safe and effective exercise.
   2. Others are exercising incorrectly and therefore are not reaping the full benefits of their program.
   3. Almost half the adult population in the United States claims to participate in some sort of physical activity. But:
      a. Slightly more than 10% report daily aerobic activity.
      b. A lower percentage engages in strength and flexibility programs.
      c. Half or more of the adult population in the United States has a weight problem.

IX. A PERSONALIZED APPROACH

A. **Because fitness and wellness needs vary significantly,all exercise and wellness prescriptions must be personalized to obtain best results.**

B. **This book provides the necessary guidelines to develop a personal lifetime program.**

C. **This book and the laboratory experiences, will help you will learn to:**
   1. Determine whether medical clearance is needed.
   2. Assess the health-related components of fitness.
   3. Write exercise prescriptions for endurance, strength, and flexibility.
   4. Conduct nutritional analyses.
   5. Write sound diet and weight-control programs.
   6. Determine cardiovascular risks and implement risk-reduction.
   7. Follow a cancer risk-reduction program.
   8. Determine your stress and implement stress management programs.
   9. Implement a smoking cessation program.
   10. Avoid chemical dependency.
   11. Learn the health consequences of sexually transmitted diseases.
   12. Discover the relationship between fitness and aging.
   13. Write objectives to improve your fitness and wellness.
   14. Learn how to chart a wellness program.
   15. Discern between myths and facts in health-related concepts.

X. U.S. HEALTH OBJECTIVES FOR THE YEAR 2000

A. **Every 10 years the U.S. Department of Health and Human Services releases a list of objectives for disease prevention and health promotion.**

B. **The Year 2000 objectives address three important points:**
   1. Personal responsibility. The need for individuals to become ever more health-conscious. Responsible and informed behaviors are the key to good health.
   2. Health benefits for all people. Lower socioeconomic conditions and poor health often are interrelated. Extending the benefits of good health to all people is crucial to the health of the nation.
   3. Health promotion and disease prevention. A shift from treatment to preventive techniques will drastically cut health care costs and help all Americans achieve a higher quality of life.

XI. WELLNESS LIFESTYLE QUESTIONNAIRE

A. **Even though exercise testing and participation is relatively safe, a person takes a small but real risk of certain bodily changes occurring during exercise testing or participation.**

B. **Before you begin an exercise program or participate in any exercise testing, you should fill out the questionnaire. If your answer to any of the questions is yes, you should see a physician before participating in a fitness program. If you have any questions regarding your current health status, consult your doctor before initiating, continuing, or increasing your level of physical activity.**

C. **Upon completion of the questionnaire, select the areas where you think you will need the most improvement. While you need to pay attention to all aspects of wellness, initially work on those lifestyle factors in which definite improvements are required.**

Instructor Activities

1. **Use overhead transparency 1-1** (master found in this manual) to focus a class discussion on the changing definitions of health through the past century. Point out that today we no longer think of health as the absence of disease nor restricted to the body.

2. **Use overhead transparency 1-2** (master found in this manual) and discuss the interdependent relationship among the various dimensions of health and wellness. Many authorities today include physical, social, emotional, intellectual, and spiritual dimensions in their health and wellness models. Some authorities also include an environmental dimension or economical dimension.

3. **Use overhead transparency 1-3** (master found in this manual) and color transparency 5 (in the Color Transparency Packet) to discuss the wellness continuum.
   1. Health as freedom from disease — a standard of mediocrity.
   2. Health as a quality of life — a standard of inspiration.

   Point out that health is often thought of as a state of being while wellness is viewed as a process that leads to our potential. Physicians play an important role in treating disease, but optimal health is based on personal lifestyle choices.

4. **Use color overhead transparency 1** (in the Color Transparency Packet) to show the deaths by selected causes in the U.S. between 1900 and 1990.

5. **Use overhead transparency 1-3** (master found in this manual) to discuss the significance of the underlying causes of disease. Compare the data on the transparency with part VI-B of this chapter outline.

6. **Divide the class into three groups**. One group should represent community health, one the medical profession, and one personal health practices. Have each group tell what they have done, what they are doing, and what they need to do as we approach the year 2000 to prevent disease and promote wellness. See part X-B in the outline for this chapter.

7. **Use color overhead transparency 4** (in the Color Transparency Packet) to identify the wellness components.

8. **Lead a class discussion** focussisng on the difference between health fitness and physical fitness standards. See part V of the chapter outline.

NOTES

WHAT IS HEALTH ?

1900

Health is the absence of disease.

1920

Health is the normal functioning of all parts of the body, complete physical fitness.

1947

Health is a state of complete physical, mental, and social well-being, not merely the absence of disease or infirmity.

1965

Health is the quality of life involving our physical, social, emotional, intellectual, and spiritual dimensions.

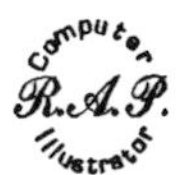

1-1

1-1

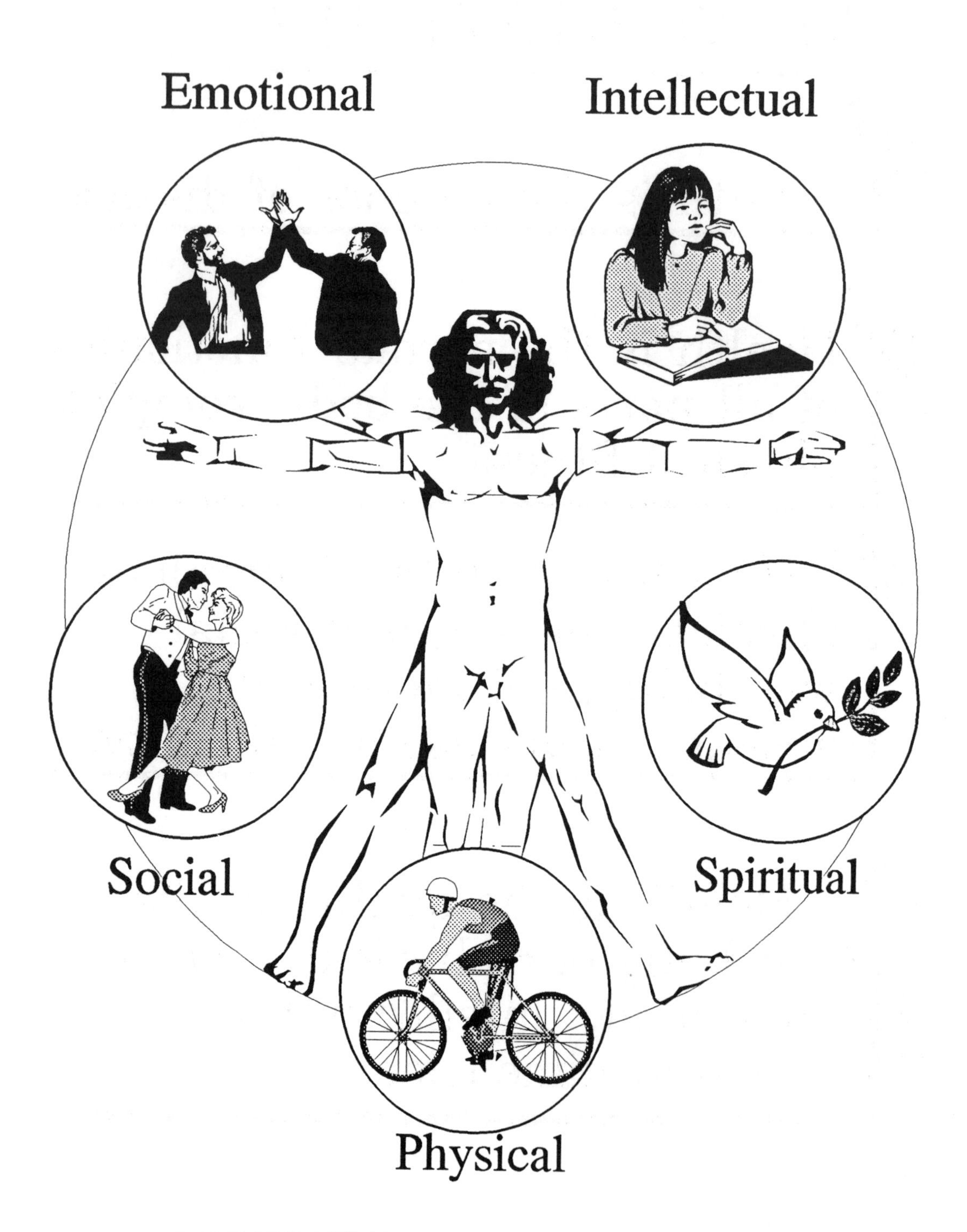
Emotional
Intellectual
Social
Spiritual
Physical

1-2

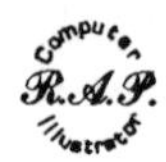
Computer
R.A.P.
Illustrator

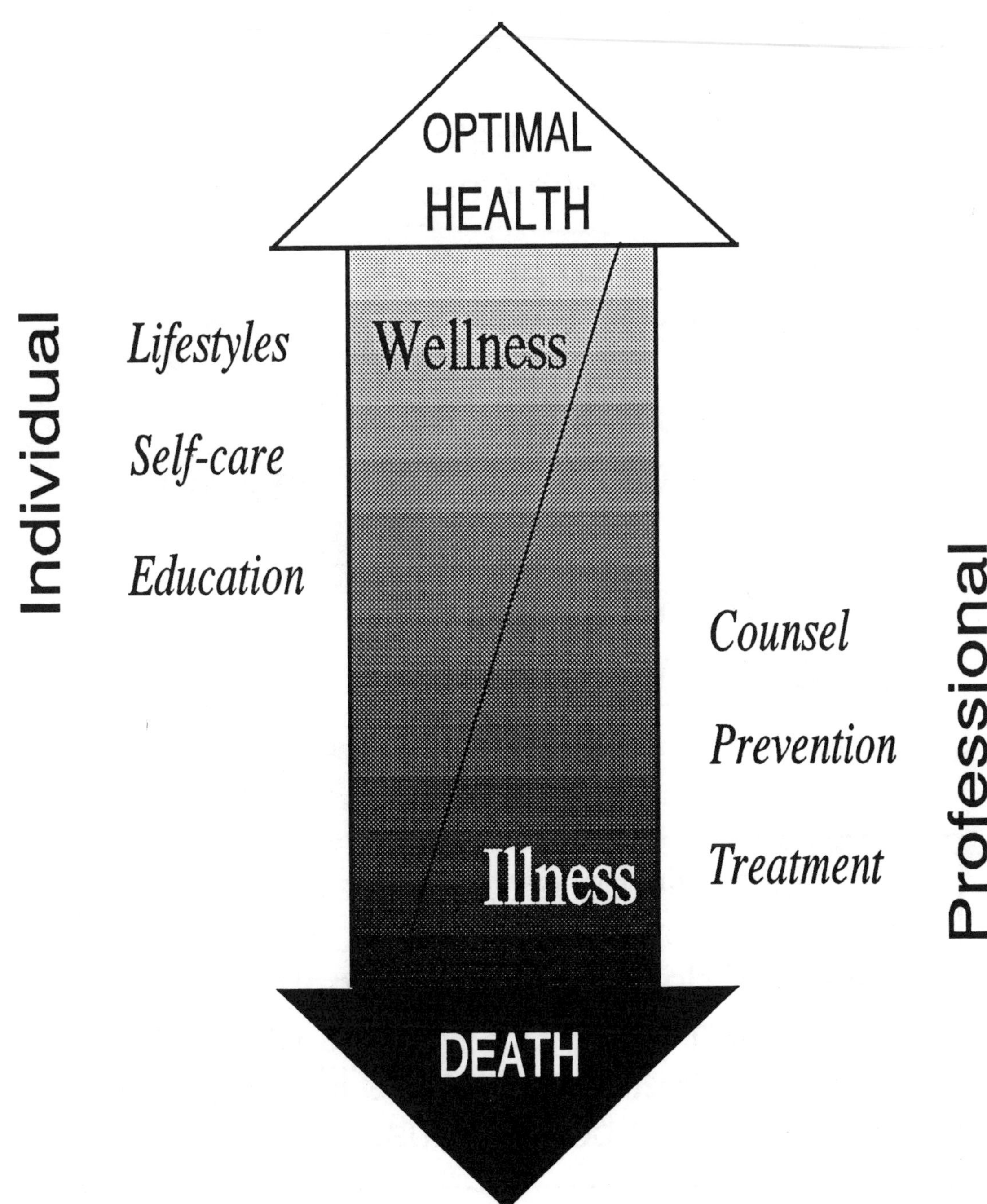
OPTIMAL
HEALTH
Individual
Lifestyles
Self-care
Education
Wellness
Counsel
Prevention
Treatment
Illness
Professional
DEATH

1-3

The Cause Of Death

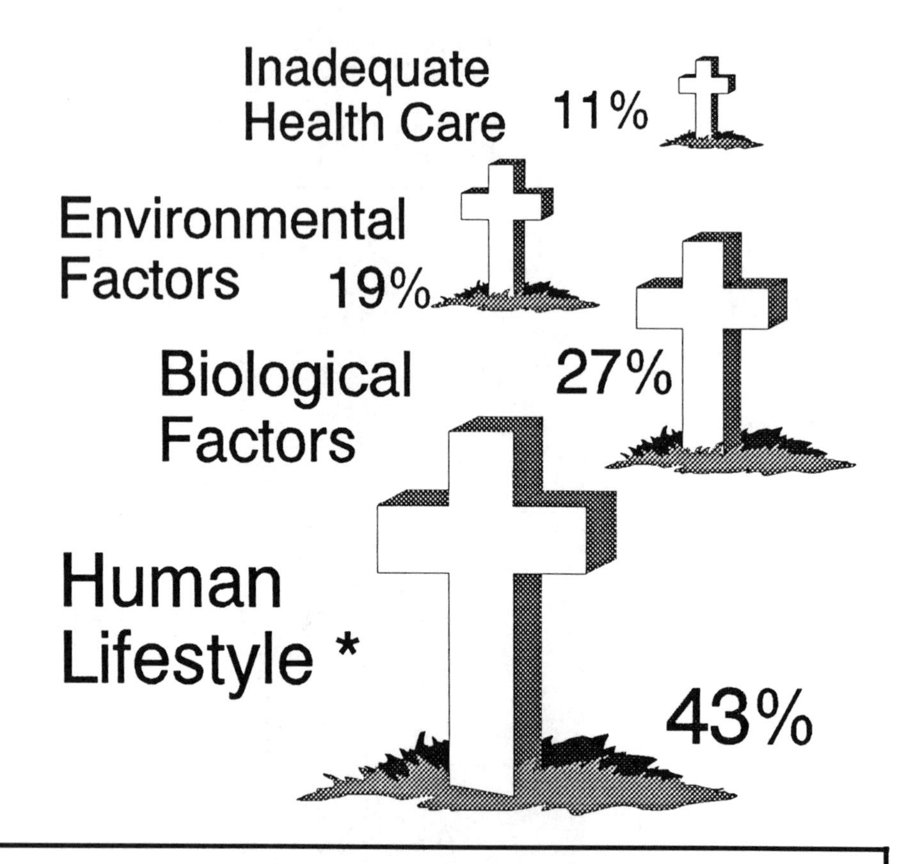

* Lifestyle consists of health-related behaviors over which the individual has personal decision-making control.

When self-imposed risks result in illness or death the victim's lifestyle is considered to be the cause.

1.4

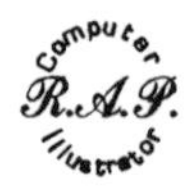

1-4

Cardiovascular Endurance Assessment

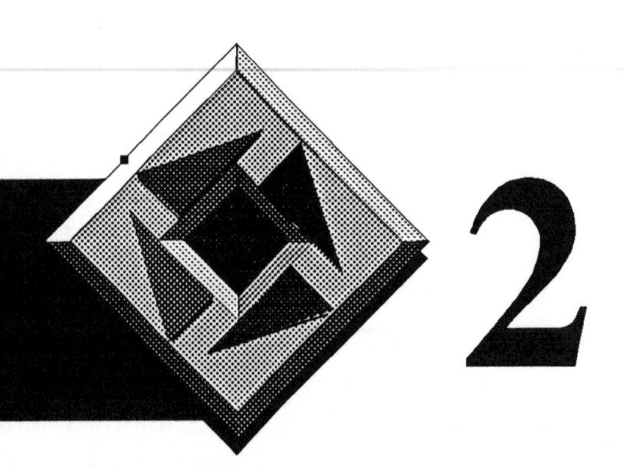

Expanded Chapter Outline

I. CARDIOVASCULAR ENDURANCE

A. Cardiovascular endurance has been defined as the ability of the lungs, heart, and blood vessels to deliver adequate amounts of oxygen to the cells to meet the demands of prolonged physical activity:

1. At the cellular level, oxygen is used to convert food substrates, primarily carbohydrates and fats, into energy necessary to conduct body functions.
2. Because the body needs more energy during physical exertion, the heart, lungs, and blood vessels have to deliver more oxygen to the cells.
3. During prolonged exercise an individual with a high level of cardiovascular endurance is able to deliver the required amount of oxygen to the tissues with relative ease.
4. The cardiovascular system of a person with a low level of endurance has to work much harder.

II. AEROBIC AND ANAEROBIC EXERCISE

A. Cardiovascular endurance activities often are called aerobic exercises.

1. The word aerobic means "with oxygen."
2. Whenever an activity requires oxygen to produce energy, it is considered an aerobic exercise.
3. Examples of cardiovascular or aerobic exercises are:
   a. walking
   b. jogging
   c. swimming
   d. cycling
   e. cross-country skiing

f. water aerobics
g. rope skipping
h. and aerobics

B. Anaerobic activities, on the other hand, are carried out "without oxygen."
1. The intensity of anaerobic exercise is so high that oxygen is not utilized to produce energy.
2. Because energy production is limited in the absence of oxygen, these activities can be carried out for only short periods (2 to 3 minutes).
3. Examples of anaerobic activities are:
   a. 100, 200, and 400 meters dash in track and field
   b. 100 meters in swimming
   c. gymnastics routines
   d. strength training

C. Only aerobic activities will help increase cardiovascular endurance.

III. IMPORTANCE OF CARDIOVASCULAR ENDURANCE

A. Physical activity is no longer a natural part of our existence.
1. In our automated world, activities that once required physical exertion are now done by machines.
2. Among the most harmful effects of modern-day technology is an increase hypokinetic (little motion) diseases, chronic conditions related to a lack of physical activity.
3. These include hypertension, heart disease, chronic low back pain, and obesity.
4. To enjoy modern technology and still expect to live life to its fullest, a lifetime exercise program must become a part of daily living.

B. There are four components of physical fitness:
1. Cardiovascular endurance is the single most important.
2. A person can get away without having large amounts of strength and flexibility but cannot do without a good cardiovascular system.
3. Cardiovascular endurance activities help maintain recommended body weight.

IV. BENEFITS OF CARDIOVASCULAR ENDURANCE TRAINING

A. Physiological adaptations from aerobic training:
1. A higher maximal oxygen uptake (Max VO2):
   a. The amount of oxygen the body is able to use during physical activity increases significantly.
   b. This allows the individual to exercise longer and at a higher rate before becoming fatigued.
   c. Small increases in Max VO2 can be observed in as few as 2 to 3 weeks of

aerobic training.

2. An increase in the oxygen-carrying capacity of the blood:
   a. As a result of training, the red blood cell count goes up.
   b. Red blood cells contain hemoglobin, which transports oxygen.
3. A decrease in resting heart rate:
   a. Resting heart rates frequently are lowered by 10 to 20 beats per minute (bpm) after only 6 to 8 weeks of training.
   b. During resting conditions, the heart ejects between 5 and 6 liters of blood per minute.
4. A lower heart rate at given workloads:
   a. A trained person has a lower heart rate response to a given task.
   b. Following several weeks of training, a given workload elicits a much lower heart rate response.
5. An increase in the number and size of the mitochondria:
   a. The energy necessary for cell function is produced in the mitochondria.
   b. Training increases the size and number of mitochondria and this increases the potential to produce energy for muscular work.
6. An increase in the number of functional capillaries:
   a. The oxygen and carbon dioxide gas exchange takes place in the capillaries.
   b. Training produces a larger number of capillaries in muscle tissue including the heart muscle.
   c. This capillarization speeds up the rate at which waste products of cell metabolism can be removed.
   d. Increased capillarization also enhances oxygen delivery capacity to the muscles.
7. Faster recovery time:
   a. Trained individuals recover more rapidly after exercising.
   b. A fit system is able to restore more quickly any internal equilibrium disrupted during exercise.
8. Lower blood pressure and blood lipid level:
   a. A regular aerobic exercise program lowers blood pressure and blood lipids such as cholesterol and triglycerides.
   b. Higher blood pressure and higher blood lipids are linked to the formation of atherosclerotic plaque, which obstructs the arteries in the heart.
   c. This decreases the risk of coronary heart disease and strokes.
9. More fat-burning enzymes:
   a. As the concentration of the enzymes increases, so does the ability to burn fat.
   b. Fat is lost primarily by burning it in muscle.

V. ASSESSMENT OF CARDIOVASCULAR ENDURANCE

A. Because all tissues of the body need oxygen to function, higher oxygen consumption indicates a more efficient cardiovascular system.

B. Cardiovascular endurance is determined by the maximal amount of oxygen (Max VO2) the human body is able to utilize per minute of physical activity.
1. This value can be expressed in:
   a. liters per minute (l/min)
   b. milliliters per kilogram per minute (ml/kg/min)
2. The most precise way to determine maximal oxygen uptake is through direct gas analysis.
   a. This type of equipment is not available in most health/fitness centers.
   b. Therefore, several alternative methods of estimating maximal oxygen uptake have been developed using limited equipment.

C. Cardiovascular endurance tests are probably safe to administer to apparently healthy individuals (those with no major coronary risk factors or symptoms).
1. However, the American College of Sports Medicine recommends that a physician be present for all maximal exercise tests on apparently healthy men over age 40 and women over age 50.
2. A maximal test is any test that requires the participant's all-out or nearly all-out effort.
3. For submaximal exercise tests a physician should be present when testing higher risk/symptomatic individuals or diseased people.
4. Five exercise tests used to assess cardiovascular fitness are introduced in this chapter:
   a. 1.5-Mile Run Test
   b. 1.0-Mile Walk Test
   c. Step Test
   d. Astrand-Ryhming Test
   e. 12-Minute Swim Test

D. Interpreting Maximal Oxygen Uptake Results:
1. After obtaining your maximal oxygen uptake, you can determine your current level of cardiovascular fitness by consulting Table 2.8.
2. Record this information in Figure 2.6 in this chapter and in your Fitness and Wellness Profile in Appendix A.

E. Exercise Readiness:
1. Before starting a cardiovascular exercise prescription, you should determine your exercise readiness.
2. Ask yourself this question, Are you willing to give exercise a try?
3. Using Figure 2.7, you can list the advantages and disadvantages of incorporating exercise into your lifestyle.
4. The information provided in Figure 2.8 then can help you answer the question: Am I ready to start an exercise program?
5. You are evaluated in four categories:
   a. mastery (self-control)
   b. attitude

c. health
d. commitment

6. The higher you score in any category the more important that reason is for you to exercise.
   a. Scores can vary from 4 to 16.
   b. If you score 12 or more points in each category, your chances of initiating and sticking to an exercise program are good.
   c. If you do not score at least 12 points in three categories, your chances of succeeding at exercise may be slim.

NOTES

Instructor Activities

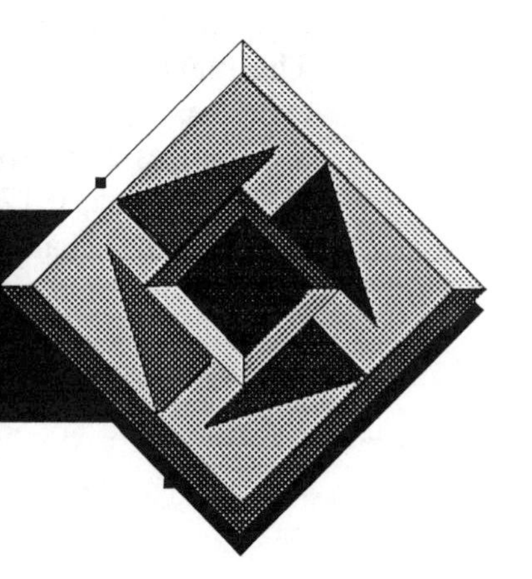

1. **On the chalkboard** write on the following statement found in the text on page 28 and ask the students to defend or refute the statement.

   Cardiovascular endurance is the most important component of health related fitness.

2. **Show overhead transparency 2-1** in this manual to explain what is meant by cardiovascular endurance.

3. **Show overhead transparency 2-2** in this manual and explain the benefits of cardiovascular endurance training.

4. **Show overhead transparencies** from the color transparency packet to show the changes in Maximum Oxygen Uptake (Max VO_2. See Tables 2.1, 2.2, and 2.3 in the text.

5. **Discuss** the assessment procedures to be used in the class for determining cardiovascular endurance.

6. **Discuss** the importance of health screening prior to physical fitness tests and exercise. Explain the circumstances that necessitate a physician's aproval before exercising and a physician's presence during screening tests. A physician should be present for a maximal exercise test. A physician should also be present for exercise tests on apparently healthy men over age 40 and women over age 50. Also discuss the importance of warming up and cooling down before and after exercising.

CARDIOVASCULAR ENDURANCE

Cardiovascular endurance has been defined as the ability of the lungs, heart, and blood vessels to deliver adequate amounts of oxygen to the cells to meet the demands of prolonged physical activity.

Oxygen is used to convert food (primarily carbohydrates and fats) into energy necessary to conduct body functions.

During prolonged exercise an individual with a high level of cardiovascular endurance is able to deliver the required amount of oxygen to the tissues with relative ease.

The cardiovascular system of a person with a low level of endurance has to work much harder.

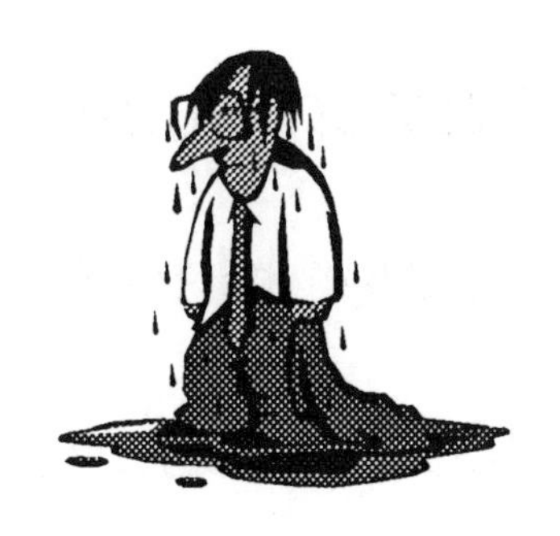

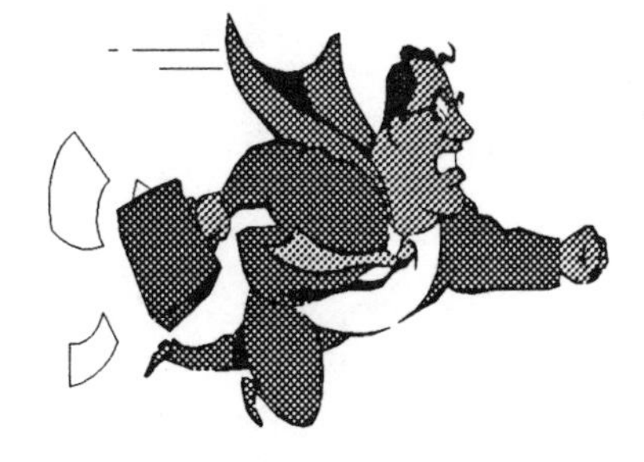

2-1

BENEFITS OF CARDIOVASCULAR ENDURANCE TRAINING

Physiological adaptations from aerobic training

1. A higher maximal oxygen uptake (Max VO_2).
2. An increase in the oxygen-carrying capacity of the blood.
3. A decrease in resting heart rate.
4. A lower heart rate at given workloads.
5. An increase in the number and size of the mitochondria (energy producing centers withen the cells).
6. An increase in the number of functional capillaries.
7. Faster recovery time.
8. Lower blood pressure and blood lipid level.
9. More fat-burning enzymes.

2-2

Cardiovascular Exercise Prescription

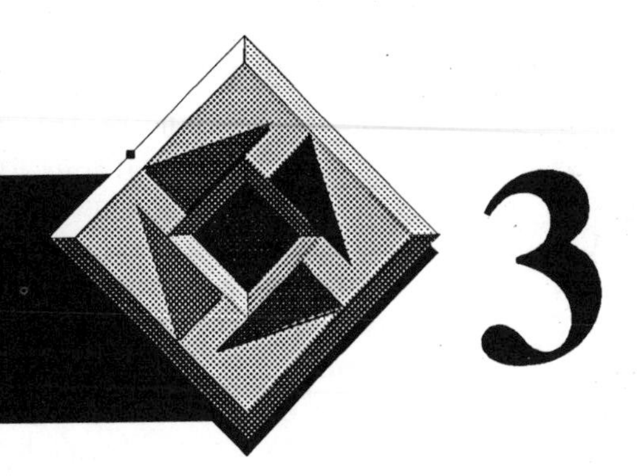

Expanded Chapter Outline

I. GUIDELINES FOR CARDIOVASCULAR EXERCISE PRESCRIPTION

A. Overloaded Principle:

1. To develop the cardiovascular system, the heart muscle has to be overloaded like any other muscle in the human body.
2. To better understand how this principle we have to be familiar with four basic principles of exercise:
   a. intensity
   b. mode
   c. duration
   d. frequency
3. Before vigorous exercise, healthy men over age 40 and women over age 50 should undergo a medical exam and a diagnostic exercise stress test.

B. Intensity of Exercise:

1. This principle refers to how hard a person has to exercise to improve cardiovascular endurance.
2. When trying to develop the cardiovascular system, intensity of exercise is the factor that perhaps is ignored most often.
3. Overloaded is accomplished with the cardiovascular system by making the heart pump faster for a certain period of time.
   a. Cardiovascular development occurs when working between 50% and 85% of heart rate reserve.
   b. The intensity of exercise can be calculated easily, and training can be monitored by checking your pulse.
   c. Determining Training Intensity of exercise or cardiovascular training:
      (1) Estimate your maximal heart rate: MHR = 220 minus age (220 - age).
      (2) Check your resting heart rate (RHR) sometime after you have been sitting quietly for 15 to 20 minutes.

(3) Determine the heart rate reserve: HRR = MHR - RHR (the number of beats between resting maximal effort).

(4) Calculate the training intensities: 50%, 70%, and 85% TI = HRR x the respective 50, 70, and 85 + RHR.

4. The cardiovascular training zone: maintain your heart rate between the 50% and 85% training intensities.
   a. The physically inactive should train around the 50% intensity during the first 4 to 6 weeks and after that between 70% and 85% training intensity.
   b. After a few weeks of training one may have a considerably lower resting heart rate (10 to 20 beats in 8 to 12 weeks). Therefore, you should recompute your target zone periodically.
5. You should monitor your exercise heart rate regularly:
   a. Start monitoring about 5 minutes into the exercise session.
   b. If the rate is too low, increase the intensity of exercise.
   c. If the rate is too high, slow down.

C. **Health Fitness Versus Physical Fitness:**
   1. Training benefits which lower the risk for cardiovascular mortality can be obtained by exercising at 50% training intensity.
   2. Achieving a high cardiovascular fitness rating (physical fitness standard) can be obtained by exercising closer to the 85% threshold.

D. **Rate of Perceived Exertion:**
   1. This is an alternative method of prescribing intensity of exercise.
   2. A person subjectively rates the perceived exertion.

E. **Mode of Exercise:**
   1. The type of exercise that develops the cardiovascular system has to be aerobic in nature:
      a. Aerobic exercise involves the major muscle groups of the body.
      b. The activity has to be rhythmic and continuous.
      c. The activity or combination of activities has to get the heart rate up to that training zone and keep it there for the duration of the exercise.
   2. Examples of these activities are:
      a. walking
      b. jogging
      c. aerobics
      d. swimming
      e. water aerobics
      f. cross-country skiing
      g. aero-belt exercise
      h. rope skipping
      i. cycling
      j. racquetball
      k. stair climbing
      l. stationary running or cycling

3. The activity you choose should be based on your personal preferences, what you most enjoy doing, and your physical limitations.

F. Duration of Exercise:

1. Train between 20 and 60 minutes per session.
2. The duration is based on how intensely a person trains.
   a. If the training is done around 85%, 20 minutes are sufficient.
   b. At 50% intensity the person should train at least 30 minutes.
   c. Unconditioned people and older adults should train at lower percentages but over a longer time.
3. Recent research indicates that three 10-minute exercise sessions per day (separated by at least 4 hours), at approximately 70% of maximal heart rate, also produce training benefits.
4. Exercise sessions always should be preceded by a 5-minute warm-up and followed by a 5-minute cool-down period.
   a. Warm-up should consist of general calisthenics, stretching exercises, or exercising at a lower intensity level than the actual target zone.
   b. The cool-down entails gradually decreasing the intensity of exercise.
      (1) Abruptly stopping causes blood to pool in the exercised body parts, diminishing the return of blood to the heart.
      (2) Less blood return can cause dizziness and faintness or even bring on cardiac abnormalities.

G. Frequency of Exercise:

1. When starting an exercise program, three to five training sessions per week are recommended.
2. When training is conducted more than 5 days a week, further improvements are minimal.
3. For individuals on a weight-loss program, 45 to 60 minute exercise sessions of low to moderate intensity are recommended.
4. As few as three 20- to-30-minute training sessions per week, on nonconsecutive days, will maintain cardiovascular fitness.

II. SPECIFIC EXERCISE CONSIDERATIONS

A. Does aerobic exercise make a person immune to heart and blood vessel disease?

1. Aerobically fit individuals as a whole have a lower incidence of cardiovascular disease.
2. A regular aerobic exercise program by itself does not offer an absolute guarantee against cardiovascular disease.
3. Many factors, including genetic predisposition, can increase the person's risk.

B. How much aerobic exercise is required to decrease the risk for cardiovascular disease?

1. It is generally recommended that 2,000 calories expended per week in physical activity yielded the lowest risk for cardiovascular disease.
2. Two thousand calories per week represents about 300 calories per daily exercise session.

C. **Is it safe to exercise during pregnancy?**

1. Women should not forsake exercise during pregnancy.
2. The woman and her personal physician should make the final decision regarding her exercise program.
3. Starting a new, strenuous exercise program during pregnancy is not recommended.
4. Women who have been exercising regularly may continue through the fourth month of pregnancy.
5. After the fourth month, walking, stationary cycling, moderate swimming, and water aerobics are indicated in conjunction with some light strengthening exercises.
6. Exercises that require a woman to lie on her back should be avoided after the fourth month.
7. Care should be taken not to exceed a body (core) temperature of 38º C (100º F).
8. Exercise heart rates should be kept below 140 beats per minute, and training sessions should be limited to 15 minutes.

D. **Does participating in exercise hinder menstruation?**

1. In some instances highly trained athletes may develop amenorrhea (stopping of menstruation) during training and competition.
2. Menstruation should not keep a woman from participating in athletics, and it will not necessarily have a negative impact on performance.

E. **Does exercise help relieve dysmenorrhea (painful menstruation)?**

1. Exercise has been shown to help relieve menstrual cramps because it improves circulation to the uterus.
2. Stretching exercises of the muscles in the pelvic region seem to reduce and prevent painful menstruation that is not the result of a disease.

F. **Does exercise offset the detrimental effects of cigarette smoking?**

1. Physical exercise often motivates toward stopping smoking, but it does not offset any ill effects of smoking.
2. Smoking greatly diminishes the ability of the blood to transport oxygen to working muscles.
3. Carbon monoxide combines much faster than oxygen with hemoglobin, decreasing the oxygen-carrying capacity of the blood.
4. Chronic smoking increases airway resistance. If a person quits smoking, exercise helps increase the functional capacity of the pulmonary system.

G. **Is exercise safe during a smog alert?**

1. People who have respiratory or cardiovascular conditions should not exercise outdoors when air quality is poor.
2. Everyone should refrain from outdoor exercise during periods of smog alert or "very poor" air quality.
   a. Exercising indoors is a safer alternative.
   b. Air quality usually is best during the early morning and late evening hours.

H. What type of clothing should a person wear during exercise?

1. Clothing should fit comfortably and allow free movement.
2. Clothes should be geared to air temperature and humidity.
   a. Exercisers should avoid nylon and rubberized materials.
   b. They should also avoid tight clothes.
3. Properly fitting shoes designed for the activity are a must.

I. How long should a person wait after a meal before exercising strenuously?

1. The length of time depends on the amount of food eaten.
2. After a large meal, wait about 2 hours before strenuous activities.
3. A walk or some other light physical activity is fine following a meal.

J. What time of day is best for exercise?

1. You can do intense exercise almost any time of the day, except within 2 hours of a heavy meal.
2. Avoid intense midday exercise on hot and humid days.
3. Moderate exercise seems to be beneficial shortly after a meal.
4. People who exercise in the morning seem to stick with it more.
5. Some prefer the lunch hour for weight control reasons.
6. Highly stressed people seem to like the evening hours.

K. Why is exercising in hot and humid conditions unsafe?

1. Much of the energy produced in exercise is converted into heat.
2. If the weather is either too hot or humidity the body has difficulty dissipating the heat.
3. There is a need for caution when exercising in hot or humid weather.

L. What should a person do to replace fluids lost during prolonged aerobic exercise?

1. The main objective of fluid replacement is to maintain the blood volume so circulation and sweating can continue at normal levels.
2. Adequate water replacement is the most important factor in preventing heat disorders.
3. Drinking about 8 ounces of cool water every 10 to 15 minutes during exercise seems to be ideal to prevent dehydration.
4. Commercial fluid replacement solutions may be helpful.
5. Sugar does not become available to the muscles until about 30 minutes after drinking a glucose solution.

M. What precautions should be taken when exercising in the cold?

1. Exercising in the cold usually does not threaten one's health.
2. Clothing for heat conservation can be selected.
3. Exercise itself increases the production of body heat.
4. It is not cold, but wind velocity that poses a threat.

III. MANAGING EXERCISE-RELATED INJURIES

A. Preventing injury during a conditioning program is essential.

B. Exercise-related injuries are common in individuals who exercise.

C. The three most common causes of injuries are:

1. rapid conditioning programs--doing too much too quickly
2. improper shoes or training surfaces
3. anatomical predisposition (body propensity)

D. Most of these injuries can be prevented through a more gradual and moderate conditioning program.

E. The best treatment always has been prevention. If an activity causes unusual discomfort something should be changed to keep it from getting worse.

1. decreasing the intensity of exercise
2. switching activities
3. substituting equipment
4. upgrading clothing (such as proper-fitting shoes)

F. In case of injury, proper treatment can avert a lengthy recovery process.

1. Acute Sports Injuries:
   a. In cases of acute injury, during the first 36 to 48 hours, the standard treatment to minimize swelling is: (ICE)
      (1) I = ice or cold application:
         (a) three to five times a day
         (b) for 15 to 20 minutes at a time
         (c) by submerging the injured area in cold water or applying ice
      (2) C = compression, or splinting (or both). An elastic bandage or wrap can be used for compression.
      (3) E = elevation of the affected body part. Elevating the body part decreases blood flow to it.
   b. After the first 36 to 48 hours, heat can be applied if swelling or inflammation has not increased.
   c. If a fracture is suspected or if doubts remain regarding the seriousness of the injury, medical evaluation should be sought.
   d. Obvious deformities suggest a fracture or dislocation.
      (1) splinting by trained personnel
      (2) cold application with an ice bag
      (3) medical attention
2. Muscle Soreness and Stiffness:
   a. Acute soreness or stiffness often sets in the first few hours after an individual begins an exercise program. This may be due to:
      (1) a lack of blood (oxygen) flow
      (2) general fatigue of the exercised muscles
   b. Delayed muscle soreness that appears several hours after exercise and lasts for two to four days may be related to
      (1) actual tiny tears in muscle tissue
      (2) tearing of connective tissue around muscles and joints

(3) Mild stretching, low-intensity exercise to stimulate blood flow, and a warm bath might help to relieve pain

c. Mild stretching before and adequately stretching after exercise helps to prevent soreness and stiffness.

d. Gradually progressing into an exercise program is important, too. A person should not attempt to do too much too quickly.

3. Exercise Intolerance:

a. When starting an exercise program, participants should stay within the heart rate target zone.

b. Exercising above this target zone may not be safe for unconditioned or high-risk individuals.

c. You do not have to exercise beyond your target zone to gain the desired cardiovascular benefits.

d. Several physical signs will tell you when you are exceeding your functional limitations. You should learn to listen to your body.

(1) a rapid or irregular heart rate
(2) difficult breathing
(3) nausea and or vomiting
(4) lightheadedness, headaches, dizziness
(5) pale or flushed skin
(6) extreme weakness, lack of energy, shakiness
(7) sore muscles or cramps
(8) tightness in the chest

e. If you notice any of these symptoms, you should seek medical attention before continuing your exercise program.

f. Recovery heart rate is another indicator of overexertion.

g. Recovery heart rate is related to fitness level.

(1) As a rule of thumb, heart rate should be below 120 beats per minute 5 minutes into recovery.
(2) If your heart rate is above 120, lower the intensity or duration of exercise, or both.
(3) If you still have a fast heart rate 5 minutes into recovery, you should consult your physician.

4. Side Stitch:

a. The cause of this sharp pain that sometimes occurs during exercise is unknown.

b. Some experts suggest that it could be related to a lack of blood flow to the respiratory muscles.

c. As you improve your physical condition, this problem will disappear unless you start training at a higher intensity.

d. If it occurs, slow down, and if it persists, stop altogether.

5. Shin Splints:

a. Are characterized by pain and irritation in the shin.

b. Usually results from one or more of the following:

(1) lack of proper and gradual conditioning
(2) doing physical activities on hard surfaces
(3) fallen arches in the feet

(4) chronic overuse
(5) muscle fatigue
(6) faulty posture
(7) improper shoes
(8) exercising when excessively overweight

c. Shin splints are managed by:
(1) removing or reducing the cause
(2) doing mild stretching exercises before and after exercise

a) ice massage for 10 minutes before and after exercise
(3) applying active heat (whirlpool and hot baths) for 15 minutes, two to three times a day.
(4) supportive taping during physical activity

6. Muscle Cramps:
a. Muscle cramps are caused by depletion of essential electrolytes or a lack of coordination between opposing muscle groups.
b. If you have a muscle cramp:
(1) first attempt to stretch the muscles involved
(2) then gently rub down the muscles
(3) and then do some mild exercises using those muscles
c. In pregnant and lactating women, muscle cramps often are related to a lack of calcium. Calcium supplements may be the answer.
d. Tight clothing also can cause cramps, by decreasing blood flow to active muscle tissue.

G. AEROBIC ACTIVITY CHOICES
1. There are a variety of activities that promote cardiovascular development.
2. You may select one or a combination of activities for your program.
3. This choice should be based on:
a. personal enjoyment
b. convenience
c. availability
4. No single activity develops total fitness.
a. For total fitness, aerobic activities should be supplemented with strength (resistance) and flexibility exercise programs.
b. Selecting a combination of aerobic activities (cross-training) can add enjoyment to the program.
5. This chapter contains information about various aerobic activities.

IV. RATING THE FITNESS BENEFITS OF AEROBIC ACTIVITIES

A. Different aerobic activities contributions to fitness various ways.

B. A summary of likely benefits of several activities is provided in Table 3.2.

V. GETTING STARTED AND ADHERING TO AN EXERCISE PROGRAM

A. The first step is to determine your exercise prescription.

B. Then the difficult part of starting and sticking to a lifetime exercise program begins.

C. One must be motivated, have lifelong dedication, and perseverance.
1. The first few weeks are probably the most difficult.
2. Soon you will develop a habit for exercise that will be deeply satisfying and will bring about a sense of self-accomplishment.

D. People have utilized the following suggestions successfully:
1. Select aerobic activities you enjoy.
2. Combine different activities.
3. Set aside a regular time for exercise.
4. Obtain the proper equipment (particularly shoes) for exercise.
5. Find a friend or group of friends to exercise with.
6. Set goals and share them with others.
7. Don't become a compulsive exerciser, learn to listen to your body.
8. Exercise in different places and facilities.
9. Keep a regular record of your activities.
10. Conduct periodic assessments.
11. If health problems arise, see a physician.

VI. A LIFETIME COMMITMENT TO FITNESS

A. The benefits of fitness can be maintained only through a regular lifetime program.
1. Exercising several hours on Saturday will not make up for doing nothing the rest of the week.
2. Exercising only once a week is unsafe for unconditioned adults.

B. The time involved in losing the benefits of exercise varies.
1. It has been estimated that the first 4 weeks of aerobic training are completely reversed in 2 consecutive weeks of physical inactivity.
2. As a rule of thumb, after 48 to 62 hours of aerobic inactivity, the cardiovascular system starts to lose some of its capacity.
3. However, if you have been exercising regularly for months or years, 2 weeks of inactivity will not hurt that much.
4. Flexibility can be maintained with two or three stretching sessions per week.
5. Strength is easily retained with just one maximal training session per week.

C. If you have to interrupt your program, you should not resume training at the same level you left off, but rather, build up gradually again.

Instructor Activities

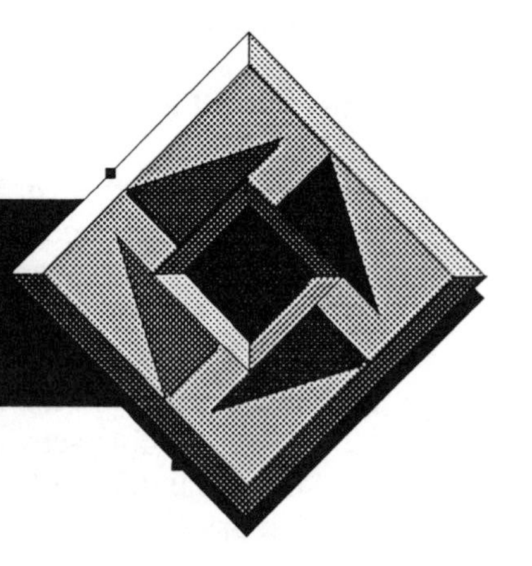

1. **Instruct the students** to take a blank sheet of paper and divide it into three sections. Ask the students to write the heading, **CURRENT EXERCISE PATTERN**, at the top of the page. Ask them to label one section **Cardiovascular Endurance**, label another section **Muscular Strength and Endurance**, and label the third section **Muscular Flexibility.** Then ask the students to list in each section what they are currently doing to develop and maintain that component of wellness. Ask the students to set this aside for now and refer back to it later. After they have completed an exercise prescription for cardiovascular health in connection with this chapter, ask them to compare their prescription with their comments on the **CURRENT EXERCISE PATTERN** sheet pertaining to cardiovascular exercise. Ask the students to save the sheet so they can make a comparison when they get to the chapters four and five strength and flexibility.

2. **Divide the class** in half with the left side of the class as group No. 1 and the right side of the class as group No. 2. Each team should select a leader and recorder. The group's task is to make a list of the major health problems that may be related to the lack of cardiovascular fitness. The group leader will field the suggestions from individuals in the group, see if the group agrees, and ask the recorder to list it on one side of the chalkboard. After a period of time, the instructor will lead the class in a comparison of the two lists.

3. **Use overhead transparency 3-1** in this manual to discuss the overload principle.

4. **Use overhead transparency 3-2** in this manual to discuss the formula for determining the intensity of the exercise. Emphasize the variables that make up the 50% to 85% range.

5. **Use transparency 11** (in the Color Transparency Packet) and discuss the *Rate of Perceived Exertion* as an alternative method of prescribing intensity.

6. **Use transparency 10** (in the color transparency packet) to discuss the typical aerobic training pattern.

7. **Discuss** the major points on the expanded chapter outline such as: Mode, Duration, and Frequency of Exercise. Also discuss specific exercise considerations and managing injuries.

OVERLOADED PRINCIPLE

To develop the cardiovascular system, the heart muscle has to be overloaded like any other muscle in the human body.

To do this you need to understand the overload principle.

The four basic components of this principles are:

Intensity

Mode

Duration

Frequency

NOTE: Before vigorous exercise, healthy men over age 40 and women over age 50 should undergo a medical exam and a diagnostic exercise stress test.

3-1

DETERMINING TRAINING INTENSITY

The intensity of exercise can be calculated.
Monitor intensity by checking your pulse.

1. Estimate your maximal heart rate:

   MHR = 220 minus age (220 - age).

2. Check your resting heart rate (RHR):
   (after resting quietly for 15 to 20 minutes.

3. Determine the heart rate reserve:
   (the number of beats between resting maximal effort).

   HRR = MHR - RHR

4. Calculate the training intensities:
   50%, 70%, and 85% *
   TI = HRR x (50, 70, or 85) + RHR.

* **The cardiovasculartrainingzone:**
The physically inactive should train around the 50% intensity during the first 4 to 6 weeks, after that between 70% to 85%.

3-2

Muscular Strength Assessment Prescription

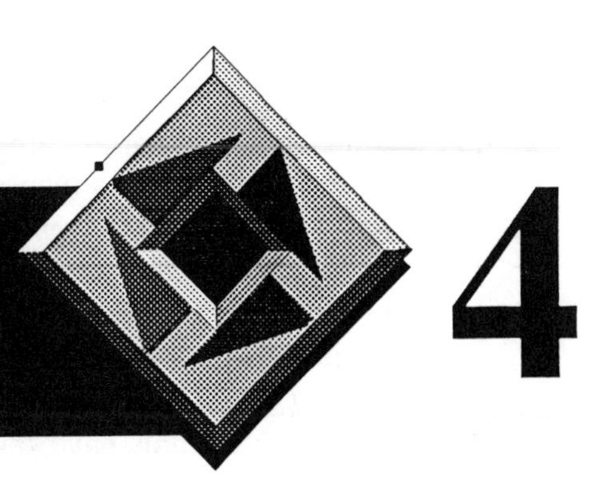

4

Expanded Chapter Outline

I. STRENGTH, HEALTH, AND INDEPENDENT LIVING

A. Many people believe that strength is only for athletes, but there is evidence that strength training enhances health:

1. Strength is a basic component of fitness and wellness and is crucial for optimal performance in daily activities.
2. Strength also is of great value in improving posture, personal appearance, and self-image.
3. Strength prepares one to meet certain emergencies in life.
4. From a health standpoint, strength helps to:
   a. maintain muscle tissue
   b. maintain a higher resting metabolism
   c. lessens the risk for injury
   d. prevent and eliminate chronic low back pain
   e. prepare for childbearing

B. For older-adults, strength might be the most important health-related component of physical fitness.

1. While cardiovascular endurance helps maintain a healthy heart, good strength levels will do more toward independent living.
2. Many older adults are confined to nursing homes because they lack sufficient strength to move about.

C. Perhaps one of the most significantbenefits of maintaininga good strength level is its relationship to human metabolism.

1. Metabolism is defined as all energy and material transformations within living cells.

2. A primary outcome of a strength training program is an increase in muscle mass or size (lean body mass), known as muscle hypertrophy.
3. Muscle tissue uses energy even at rest. In contrast, fatty tissue uses very little energy.
4. As muscle size increases, so does the resting metabolism.
   a. Estimates indicate that each additional pound of muscle tissue increases resting metabolism by 30 to 50 calories per day.
   b. If two individuals have the same weight, but have different amounts of muscle mass, the one with more muscle can ingest more calories without gaining weight.

D. Loss of lean tissue is thought to be the main reason for the decrease in metabolism as people grow older.

1. Contrary to some beliefs, metabolism does not have to slow down significantly with aging.
2. It is not so much that metabolism slows down; it's that we slow down.
3. Lean body mass decreases with sedentary living, which, in turn, slows down the resting metabolic rate.
4. If people continue eating at the same rate as their activity decreases, body fat increases.

E. Another benefit of strength training is a decrease in fatty tissue around the muscle fibers.

1. The decrease in fatty tissue often is greater than the amount of muscle hypertrophy: therefore, one loses inches but not body weight.
2. Because muscle tissue is more dense than fatty tissue, people often become discouraged because they don't lose weight.
3. They can offset this discouragement by recognizing the improvement in composition.

II. STRENGTH DIFFERENCES BETWEEN SEXES

A. The increase in muscle mass commonly seen in men who exercise does not take place in women who exercise.

1. Endocrinological differences between men and women do not allow women to achieve the muscle hypertrophy (size) that men do.
2. Men have more muscle fibers and this gives men more potential for hypertrophy.

B. Masculinityand femininityare established by genetic inheritance, not by the amount of physical activity.

1. Variations in the extent of masculinity and femininity are determined by individual differences in hormonal secretions.
2. Women with a natural physical advantage are more inclined to participate in sports. As a result, people may falsely associate participation in sports and strength

training with large muscle size.
3. As more women participate in sports, the myth will abate.

C. **In recent years improved body appearance has become the rule rather than the exception for women who participate in strength training programs.**

D. **Women body builders appear to develop heavy musculature.**
1. Does weight training masculinize women?
2. The objective of their training is to "pump" extra blood into the muscles, which makes the muscles appear much bigger than they are in a resting condition.
3. The muscles can remain filled with blood, appearing measurably larger for several hours after completing the training session.
4. In real life, these women are not as muscular as they seem when they are "pumped up" for a contest.

E. **A controversial point in the sport of body building is the use of anabolic steroids and human growth hormones.**
1. Anabolic steroids are synthetic versions of the male sex hormone testosterone, which promotes muscle development and hypertrophy.
2. About 80% of women body builders have used steroids to develop muscle mass.
3. These hormones, however, produce detrimental and undesirable side effects:
   a. hypertension
   b. fluid retention
   c. decreased breast size
   d. deepening of the voice
   e. facial whiskers body hair

III. ASSESSMENT OF MUSCULAR STRENGTH AND ENDURANCE

A. **Although muscular strength and endurance are interrelated, they differ in the following ways:**
1. Strength is defined as the ability to exert maximum force against resistance.
2. Endurance is the ability of a muscle to exert submaximal force repeatedly over time.
3. Muscular endurance depends on muscular strength and to a much lesser extent on cardiovascular endurance.

B. **Strength tests have been designed to measure muscular strength, muscular endurance, or a combination of the two.**
1. Muscular strength usually is determined by the maximal amount of resistance an individual is able to lift in a single effort.
2. Muscular endurance commonly is established by the number of repetitions an individual can perform against a submaximal resistance.
3. In strength testing several body sites should be tested.
   a. Muscular Strength and Endurance Test

   b. Muscular Endurance Test
   c. Strength-To-Body Weight Ratio Test
   d. Hand Grip Test
4. Recording Your Strength Fitness Category

IV. STRENGTH TRAINING PRESCRIPTION

A. Muscle cells increase and decrease their capacity to exert force according to the demands placed upon the muscular system.

B. If muscle cells are overloaded beyond their normal use, such as in strength training programs, the cells increase in size (hypertrophy) and strength.

C. If the demands placed on the muscle cells decrease, the cells decrease in size (atrophy) and lose strength.

V. FACTORS THAT AFFECT STRENGTH

A. Several physiological factors are related to muscle contraction and subsequent strength gains:

1. Neural Stimulation:
   a. Motor neurons branch and attach to multiple muscle fibers.
   b. Stimulation of a motor neuron causes the muscle fibers to contract maximally or not at all.
   c. The number of fibers innervated and the frequency of their stimulation determine the strength of the muscle contraction.
2. Types of Fiber:
   a. Slow-twitch or red fibers have a greater capacity for aerobic work.
   b. Fast-twitch or white fibers have a greater capacity for anaerobic work (quick and powerful movements commonly used in strength training activities).
   c. The proportion of slow- and fast-twitch fibers is determined genetically.
   d. Training increases the functional capacity of both types of fiber.
3. Overload Principle:
   a. Strength gains are achieved through increased ability of individual muscle fibers to generate a stronger contraction.
   b. Strength gains are also achieved by engaging a greater proportion of the total available fibers in each contraction.
   c. These two factors combine in the overload principle.
      (1) for strength to improve, the demands placed on the muscle must be increased systematically and progressively over time
      (2) the resistance must be of a magnitude significant enough to cause physiologic adaptation
      (3) strength training also is called progressive resistance training
4. Specificity of Training:

a. The principle of specificity of training holds that, for a muscle to increase in strength or endurance, the training program must be specific to obtain the desired effects.
b. In like manner, to increase static (isometric) versus dynamic (isotonic) strength, an individual must use static against dynamic training to achieve the desired results.

VI. PRINCIPLES INVOLVED IN STRENGTH TRAINING

A. Mode of Training:

1. Two basic types of training methods are used to improve strength: isometric (static) and isotonic (dynamic):
    a. Isometric training refers to a muscle contraction that produces little or no movement such as pushing or pulling against an immovable object.
    b. Isotonic training refers to a muscle contraction with movement, such as extending the knees with resistance or weight on the ankles.
2. The mode of training an individual selects depends mainly on the type of equipment available and the specific objective of the training.
3. Isotonic training is the most popular mode for strength training:
    a. Most daily activities are isotonic in nature.
    b. Isotonic training programs can be conducted with or without weights.
        (1) With free weights, resistance machines, or isokinetic equipment.
        (2) Without weights such as pull-ups or push-ups.
    c. In isotonic training a constant resistance is moved through a joint's full range of motion.
        (1) The greatest resistance that can be lifted equals the maximum weight that can be moved at the weakest angle of the joint.
        (2) This is because of changes in muscle length and angle of pull as the joint moves through its range of motion.
    d. As isotonic strength training became more popular, new strength training machines were developed.
        (1) Isokinetic and variable-resistance training provide differing amounts of resistance to overloading the muscle group maximally through the entire range of motion.
        (2) With isokinetic training the speed of the muscle contraction is kept constant.
4. Isometric training does not require much equipment:
    a. Strength gains are specific to the angle of muscle contraction.
    b. This type of training is beneficial in a sport such as gymnastics.
    c. Research, however, has not shown this type of training to be more effective than isotonic training.

B. Resistance:

1. Resistance in strength training is the equivalent of intensity in cardiovascular

exercise.

2. The amount of resistance, or weight lifted, depends on whether one is trying to develop muscular strength or muscular endurance.
    a. To stimulate strength development, a resistance of 80% of the maximum capacity is recommended (1 RM).
    b. Less than 80% will help increase muscular endurance rather than strength.
3. One should perform between 3 and 12 repetitions maximum for adequate strength gains (3 to 12 RM).
    a. Once the person can lift weight more than 12 times, the resistance should be increased by 5 to 10 pounds.
    b. The person should then build up to 12 repetitions again.
    c. Working near 1 RM produces the greatest strength gains.
    d. However, working constantly near 1 RM increases the risk for injury.
    e. Working around 10 repetitions maximum seems to produce the best results in terms of muscular hypertrophy.
4. Body builders tend to work with moderate resistance (60% of max.), but with more (perhaps 20) repetitions.
    a. This promotes blood flow to the muscles, "pumping up the muscles."
    b. This makes the muscles look much larger than they are in a relaxed state.

C. **Sets:**

1. A set has been defined as the number of repetitions performed for a given exercise.
    a. A person lifting a certain weight eight times has performed one set of eight repetitions.
    b. When working with 8 to 12 repetitions maximum, three sets per exercise are recommended.
2. Because of the characteristics of muscle fiber, the number of sets that can be done is limited.
    a. As the number of sets increases, so does the amount of muscle fatigue and subsequent recovery time required.
    b. Therefore, strength gains may be lessened by performing too many sets.
3. A recommended program for beginners in their first year of training is three heavy sets.
    a. The first heavy set should be preceded by one or two light warm-up sets using about 50% of the 1 RM.
    b. No warm-up sets are necessary for subsequent sets using the same muscle group.
4. To avoid muscle soreness and stiffness, new participants ought to build up gradually to the three sets of maximal repetitions.
    a. The first day do only one set of each exercise with a lighter resistance.
    b. On the second day do two sets of each exercise, the first light and the second with regular (heavy) resistance.
    c. On the third day, do three sets, one light and two heavy.
    d. After that, a person should be able to do all three heavy sets.

5. The time necessary to recover between sets is approximately 3 minutes.
    a. Ten seconds of maximal exercise pretty much depletes the energy stores in the exercised muscle(s).
    b. These stores are replenished in about 3 minutes of recovery.
6. The exercise program will be more time-effective by alternating two or three exercises that require different muscle groups.
    a. A person can proceed to an exercise for a second muscle group while they are recovering from exercising the first muscle group.
    b. Then the person can work on a third muscle group before returning to the first muscle group.
    c. For example, bench press, leg extensions, and sit-ups may be combined.

D. **Frequency of Training:**
1. Strength training should be done through either:
    a. A total body workout three times a week
    b. A split body routine more frequently
        (1) upper body one day
        (2) lower body the next day
    c. Muscles should be rested for 2 or 3 days to allow recovery.
    d. If not completely recovered, the person will not gain the full benefits.
    e. The person should do fewer sets than in the previous workout.
2. 8 weeks of consecutive training is necessary to achieve significant strength gains.
3. After achieving an ideal strength level, one training session per week will be sufficient to maintain the new strength level.

VII. PLYOMETRICS

A. **Plyometric exercise is defined best as training incorporating speed and strength to enhance explosiveness.**
1. The objective is to generate the greatest amount of force in the shortest time.
2. Strength, speed, and explosiveness are all crucial for success in athletics.
3. Greater increases in speed and explosiveness are thought possible with plyometric training.

B. **One plyometric exercise involves jumping off and back onto a box, attempting to rebound as quickly as possible on each jump.**
1. Box heights are increased progressively from about 12" to 22".
2. The bounding action attempts to take advantage of the stretch-recoil and stretch reflex characteristics of muscle.
3. The rapid stretch applied to the muscle during ground contact is thought to augment muscle contraction, leading to more explosiveness.

C. **Push-ups with a forceful extension of the arms is a plyometrics exercise used for strengthening upper body muscles.**

D. **Plyometric training has a higher risk for injuries compared to conventional modes of**

progressive resistance training.

VIII. STRENGTH TRAINING EXERCISES

A. **The three strength training programs introduced next provide a complete body workout:**
   1. The first requires only a minimum of equipment:
      a. Your body weight is used as the primary resistance for most exercises.
      b. A few exercises call for a friend's help or some basic implements from around your house.
   2. The second program requires a machine such as the Universal Gym:
      a. These exercises can be conducted on either fixed-resistance or variable-resistance equipment.
      b. Many of these exercises also can be performed with free weights.
   3. The third program requires a variable resistance machine such as the Nautilus.

IX. SETTING UP YOUR OWN STRENGTH TRAINING PROGRAM

A. **You can choose one of the three training programs outlined in this chapter depending on the facilities available.**

B. **The resistance and the number of repetitions you use should be based on whether you want to increase muscular strength or muscular endurance.**
   1. Do up to 12 repetitions maximum for strength gains.
   2. Do more than 12 for muscular endurance.
   3. If you are training for health fitness, about 12 repetitions for each exercise you will obtain good strength gains and yet be close to the endurance threshold.
   4. The only exercise that calls for more than 12 repetitions is the abdominal group which may require up to 20 repetitions.

C. **Three training sessions per week on nonconsecutive days is recommended.**

D. **Three sets are enough.**

E. **If time is a concern in completing a strength training exercise program, the American College of Sports Medicine recommends as a minimum:**
   1. 8 to 10 exercises involving the major muscle groups of the body
   2. one set of 8 to 12 repetitions performed to near fatigue
   3. conducted twice a week

Instructor Activities

1. **Use transparency 4** (in the color transparency packet) to identify the wellness components. Then point out that in this lesson the wellness component is muscular strength.

2. **Use transparency 4-1** (in this manual) to discuss distinguish between muscular strength and muscular endurance. Also distinguish between hypertrophy and atrophy.

3. **Use transparency 4-2** (in this manual) to discuss the benefits muscular strength. Ask the students to share examples.

4. **Use transparencies** from the color transparency packet as they apply to this lesson.

5. **Discuss** the benefits of maintaining a good strength level is its relationship to human metabolism and weight management.

6. **Ask the Students** to compare their comments on the **CURRENT EXERCISE PATTERN** sheet from the last chapter with their muscular strength prescription developed in this lesson.

STRENGTH

Muscularstrength-- the ability to exert maximum force against resistance.

Muscularendurance-- the ability of a muscle to exert sub-maximal force repeatedly over a period of time.

The capacity of muscle cells to exert force increases and decreases according to the demands placed upon the muscular system.

A. When muscle cells are overloaded beyond their normal use, the cells increase in size **(hypertrophy)**and strength.

B. If the demands placed on the muscle cells decrease, the cells decrease in size **(atrophy)** and lose strength.

4-1

SIGNIFICANCE OF STRENGTH

1. For optimal performance in daily tasks and recreational activities.
2. To improve personal appearance and self-image.
3. To lessen the risk of injury.
4. To cope with emergency situations in life.
5. To contribute to weight control.
6. To enhance overall health and well-being.
7. To maintain good metabolism.

4-2

PRINCIPLES OF STRENGTH TRAINING

Mode of Training:

isometric (static) or isotonic (dynamic
equipment and objective

Resistance:

The equivalent of intensity.
80% of the maximum capacity (1 RM).

Sets:

The number of exercise periods.
Example: three sets of 8 to 12 repetitions.

Frequencyof Training:

A total body workout three times a week
or
A split body routine more frequently

Rrecovery:

Muscles should be rested for 2 or 3 days.

4-3

Muscular Flexibility Assessment Prescription

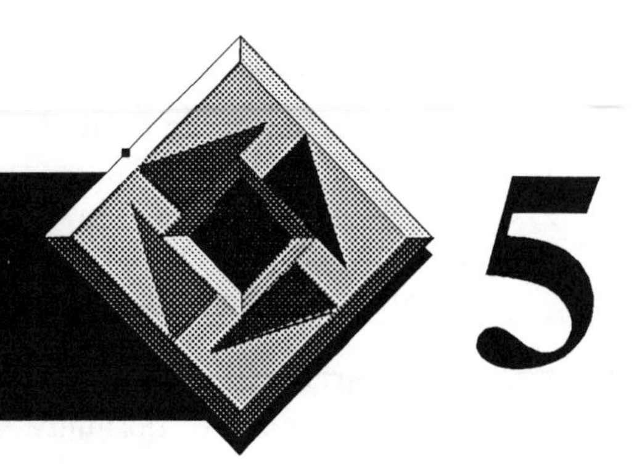

5

Expanded Chapter Outline

I. FLEXIBILITY

A. Flexibility is defined as the ability of a joint to move freely through its full range of motion.

1. Injuries due to improper body mechanics often are the result of poor flexibility:
   a. Approximately 80% of all low back problems are the result of inflexible and weak muscles.
   b. This backache syndrome costs American industry more than $1 billion each year in lost productivity.
   c. It costs industry an extra $225 million in worker's compensation.
2. Health-care professionals generally have underestimated and overlooked the contribution of flexibility to overall fitness.

B. Improving and maintaining good range of motion in the joints is important to enhance the quality of life.

C. Participating in a regular flexibility program will:

1. help a person maintain good joint mobility
2. increase resistance to muscle injury and soreness
3. prevent low-back and other spinal column problems
4. improve and maintain good postural alignment
5. promote proper and graceful body movement
6. improve personal appearance and self-image
7. help to develop and maintain motor skills throughout life

D. Flexibility exercises have been prescribed to treat:

1. dysmenorrhea or painful menstruation
2. general neuromuscular tension and stress

E. Stretching exercises in the form of calisthenics are helpful:

1. as warm-up routines to prepare for more vigorous exercises
2. as cool-down routines following exercise
   a. fatigued muscles fibers tend to contract and become short.
   b. stretching helps them reestablish their normal resting length.

F. Good range of motion is critical in older life:

1. Because of a lack of flexibility, some older adults are unable to perform simple daily tasks.
2. Many older adults do not turn their head or rotate their trunk to look over their shoulder but, rather, step around to see behind them.
3. Their enjoyment from physical activity can be hampered severely by lack of good range of motion.
4. A vicious circle then ensues, because the condition usually worsens with further inactivity.
5. A simple stretching program can alleviate or prevent this problem and help people return to an exercise program.

II. FACTORS AFFECTING FLEXIBILITY

A. Total range of motion around a joint is highly specific:

1. It varies from one joint to another (hip, trunk, shoulder).
2. It also varies from one individual to the next.
3. Muscular flexibility relates to genetic factors.
4. It also relates to physical activity.
5. Other factors influence range of motion about a joint:
   a. joint structure
   b. ligaments, tendons, muscles, and skin
   c. tissue injury
   d. adipose tissue (fat)
   e. body temperature
   f. age and sex

B. Because of the specificity of flexibility, it is difficult to indicating what constitutes an ideal level of flexibility:

1. The range of motion about a given joint can be extended through stretching exercises:
   a. Plastic elongation is the permanent lengthening of soft tissue through slow-sustained stretching exercises.
   b. Elastic elongation is the temporary lengthening of soft tissue through stretching exercises.
2. Changes in muscle temperature can increase or decrease flexibility by as much as 20%:
   a. Properly warmed-up individuals have better flexibility than non-warmed-up

people.
b. Cool temperatures have the opposite effect, impeding joint range of motion.
c. Because aerobic activities raise body temperature and facilitate plastic elongation many people prefer to do their stretching exercises after the aerobic phase of their workout.
3. A large amount of adipose (fat) tissue in and around joints and muscle tissue increases resistance to movement and hampers joint mobility.
4. On the average, women have more flexibility than men do, and they seem to retain this advantage throughout life.
5. Aging does decrease the extensibility of soft tissue, though, resulting in less flexibility in both sexes.

C. The two most significant contributors to lower flexibility levels are sedentary living and lack of exercise.
1. With less physical activity:
   a. muscles lose their elasticity
   b. tendons and ligaments tighten and shorten
   c. deposits of adipose tissue increase
2. Injury to muscle tissue and tight skin from excessive scar tissue has a negative effect on joint range of motion.

III. ASSESSMENT OF FLEXIBILITY

A. Most flexibility tests are specific to certain sports and are not practical for the general population.
1. Most health/fitness centers have relied on the Sit-and-Reach Test as an indicator of overall flexibility:
   a. This test measures flexibility of the hamstring muscles (back of the thigh) and, to a lesser extent, the lower back muscles.
   b. The test used here has been modified from the traditional Sit-and-Reach test.
   c. With the traditional test people with long arms and short legs or with short arms and long legs have an advantage.
2. Total Body Rotation Test and the Shoulder Rotation Test are indicators of everyday movements such as reaching, bending, and turning.

B. Flexibility is joint-specific and flexibility in one joint does not indicate flexibility in other joints:
1. The procedures and norms for the battery of flexibility tests are described in Figures 5.1 through 5.3 and Tables 5.1 through 5.3.
2. For the flexibility profile you should take all three tests.
3. After obtaining your scores and percentile ranks for each test, you can determine the fitness category.

IV. INTERPRETING FLEXIBILITY TEST RESULTS

A. You can determine the fitness category for each test using the guidelines given in Table 5.4. You can use Figure 5.4 to record your flexibility fitness results.

B. The overall flexibility fitness classification is obtained by computing an average percentile rank from all three tests and using the guidelines given in Table 5.4.

C. You also should record your overall flexibility results in the fitness and wellness profile given in Appendix A.

V. PRINCIPLES OF MUSCULAR FLEXIBILITY PRESCRIPTION

A. The range of joint mobility can be increased and maintained through a regular flexibility exercise program:

1. A comprehensive stretching program should include all body parts and follow the basic guidelines for flexibility development.
2. The overload and specificity of training principles discussed in conjunction with strength development apply as well to the development of muscular flexibility.
3. To increase the total range of motion of a joint, the muscles surrounding that joint have to be stretched progressively beyond their accustomed length.
4. The principles of mode, intensity, repetitions, and frequency of exercise also can be applied to flexibility programs.

B. Mode of Training

1. Three modes of stretching exercises can increase flexibility:
   a. Ballistic stretching
   b. Slow-sustained stretching
   c. Proprioceptive neuromuscular facilitation stretching
2. All three types of stretching are effective in improving flexibility, each technique has certain advantages.
3. Precautions must be taken not to overstretch ligaments.
   a. They may undergo plastic or permanent elongation.
   b. This leads to excessively loose joints and increasing the risk for injuries.
   c. Most authorities, therefore, do not recommend ballistic exercises for development of flexibility.
4. The slow-sustained stretching techniques cause little pain and are safer.
   a. muscles are lengthened gradually through a joint's complete range of motion
   b. the final position is held for a few seconds
5. Proprioceptive neuromuscular facilitation (PNF) stretching has become more popular in the last few years.
   a. This technique, based on a "contract and relax" method, requires the assistance of another person.

b. The person assisting provides initial force by pushing slowly, but does not cover the entire range of motion.
c. The person being stretched then applies force in the opposite direction of the stretch, against the assistant.
d. After 4 or 5 seconds of isometric contraction, the muscle being stretched is relaxed completely.
e. The isometric contraction is repeated for another 4 or 5 seconds, the assistant then increases the degree of stretch slowly to a greater angle.
f. Following this the muscle is relaxed again.
g. The process is repeated two to five times, until the exerciser feels mild discomfort.
h. On the last trial the final stretched position should be held for several seconds.

C. **Intensity of Exercise:**
1. The intensity, or degree of stretch, when doing flexibility exercises, should be only to a point of mild discomfort, not to the point of pain.
2. After completing the stretch, the body part is brought back gradually to the starting point.

D. **Repetitions:**
1. The time required for a flexibility development session is based on the number of repetitions and the length of time each repetition.
2. The general recommendation is that each exercise be done four or five times, holding the final position each time about 20 seconds.
3. As flexibility increases, a person can gradually increase the time each repetition is held, to a maximum of one minute.
4. Individuals who are susceptible to flexibility injuries, however, should limit each stretch to 20 seconds.

E. **Frequency of Exercise:**
1. In the early stages of the program flexibility exercises should be conducted five to six times a week.
2. After a minimum of 6 to 8 weeks of almost daily stretching, flexibility levels can be maintained with only two or three sessions per week doing about three repetitions of 10 to 15 seconds each.

VI. WHEN TO STRETCH?

A. **Many people do not differentiate a warm-up from stretching:**
1. Warming up means starting a workout slowly.
2. Stretching implies movement of joints through their range of motion.

B. **Before performing flexibility exercises, the muscles should be warmed up properly:**
1. Failing to warm up increases the risk for muscle pulls and tears.

2. Individuals who stretch before workouts without a warm-up have a higher rate of injuries than those who do not stretch at all.

C. A good time to do flexibilityexercises is after aerobic workouts:
1. Higher body temperature helps to increase joint range of motion.
2. A fatigued muscle tends to shorten and experience soreness and spasms unless stretching exercises help reestablish their normal resting length.

VII. FLEXIBILITY EXERCISES

A. To improve body flexibility,each major muscle group should be subjected to at least one stretching exercise.
B. A complete flexibilityworkout will last between 15 and 30 minutes.

VIII. PREVENTING AND REHABILITATING LOW BACK PAIN

A. Most people have low back pain at some point in their life.
1. An estimated 75 million Americans currently suffer from chronic low back pain each year.
2. About 80% of the time, backache syndrome is preventable.
3. Low back pain is caused by:
   a. physical inactivity (the most common reason)
   b. poor postural habits and body mechanics
   c. excessive body weight

B. Incorrect posture and poor mechanics increase strain in the lower-back:
1. This tilt puts extra pressure on the spinal vertebrae, causing pain in the lower back.

2. Accumulation of fat around the midsection of the body contributes to the forward tilt of the pelvis, which further aggravates the condition.

C. Low back pain can be reduced greatly by includingsome specific stretchingand strengtheningexercises in the regular fitness program.

D. If the pain is severe and persistseven at rest, consult a physician.
1. The physician can rule out any disc damage.
2. The physician may prescribe proper bed rest.
   a. Put several pillows under the knees for leg support.
   b. This position helps release muscle spasms by stretching the muscles involved.
   c. A physician may prescribe a muscle relaxant or anti-inflammatory medication (or both).

E. Once a person is pain-free in the resting state, exercise may be used to stretch the tight muscles and strengthen the weak ones.

1. Several exercises help prevent and rehabilitate the backache syndrome.
2. These exercises can be done twice or more daily when a person has back pain.
3. Doing these exercises three to four times a week is enough to prevent the syndrome.

Instructor Activities

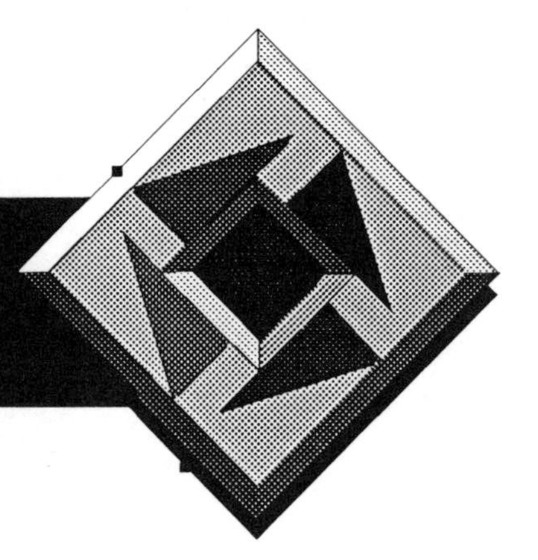

1. **Discuss** the reasons why individuals have varying degrees of flexibility. Genetics plays a critical in determining body flexibility.

2. **Discuss** the reasons why a person has varying degrees of flexibility from one joint to another. Range of motion is highly specific to each body part.

3. **Discuss** the reasons why flexibility differs from one person to another depending on their history of activity. The range of joint mobility can be increased and maintained or reduced and lost.

4. **Assign** the students to visit an area in the community where elderly people are taking part in a variety of activities and observe the difference in their flexibility. Flexibility may be the most critical component of fitness for the elderly.

5. **Discuss** the precautions that must be taken during flexibility exercises to prevent overstretch of ligaments. Emphasize the importance of a proper warmup. Discuss the selection of exercise mode. Most authorities, do not recommend ballistic exercises for flexibility.

6. **Use transparency 5-1** in this manual to discuss guideline for flexibility development.

7. **Use transparency 5-2** in this manual to discuss how to design a flexibility program.

8. **Use transparencies** from the color transparency packet as they apply to this lesson.

GUIDELINES FOR FLEXIBILITY DEVELOPMENT

MODE

ballistic stretching
slow-sustained stretching
proprioceptive neuromuscular facilitation stretching

INTENSITY

The muscles always should be warmed up.
Sketch only to a point of mild discomfort.
Hold and relax the muscles being stretched.
Bring back to the starting point gradually.

REPETITIONS

Do each exercise four or five times.
At first, hold the final position for about 10 seconds.
Later, it can be held for a minute.

FREQUENCY

At first, five to six times a week.
Later, (6 to 8 weeks) two or three times a week.

5-1

DESIGNING A FLEXIBILITY PROGRAM

Involve each major muscle group.

Use at least one stretching exercise for each muscle group.

Use the joint's full range of motion.

Use about 3 repetitions of 10 to 15 seconds each.

A complete workout will last between 15 and 30 minutes.

At first, do a complete workout five to six times a week.

After six to eight weeks. a complete workout two or three times a week is sufficient.

5-2

Body Compowition Assessment

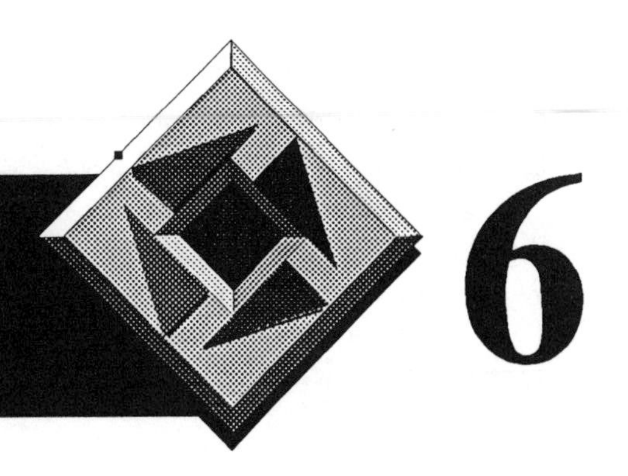

6

Expanded Chapter Outline

I. OBESITY

A. Obesity is a health hazard of epidemic proportions in most developed countries around the world:

1. An estimated 35% of the adult population is obese.
2. 65% of adults in the U.S. are over recommended body weight.
3. This problem seems to be getting worse.

B. Obesity has been associated with several serious health problems:

1. diseases of the cardiovascular system:
    a. coronary heart disease
    b. hypertension
    c. congestive heart failure
    d. high levels of blood lipids
    e. atherosclerosis
    f. strokes
    g. thromboembolitic disease
2. several types of cancer:
    a. colon
    b. rectum
    c. prostate
    d. gallbladder
    e. breast
    f. uterus
    g. ovaries
3. diabetes
4. osteoarthritis

5. varicose veins
6. ruptured intervertebral discs
7. gallstones
8. gout
9. respiratory insufficiency
10. complications during pregnancy and delivery
11. psychological maladjustment
12. accidental deaths

C. **The pressure to attain thinness contributes to the increase in the number of people who develop eating disorders--anorexia nervosa and bulimia.**

D. **Extreme weight loss is associated with a number of serious health problems:**
1. heart damage
2. gastrointestinal problems
3. shrinkage of internal organs
4. immune system abnormalities
5. disorders of the reproductive system
6. loss of muscle tissue
7. damage to the nervous system
8. death

II. WHAT DOES "BODY COMPOSITION" MEAN?

A. **The human body consists of fat and non-fat components:**
1. The fat component usually is called fat mass or percent body fat.
2. The nonfat component is termed lean body mass.

B. **We once relied on height/weight charts to determine recommended weight.**

C. **We now know that these tables can be highly inaccurate.**
1. With height/weight charts a person can be overweight, according to the charts, yet have a low percent of body fat.
2. Or a person can be underweight, according to the charts, yet have a high percent of body fat.

D. **A much better way to determine body composition.**

E. **Find out what percent of total body weight is fat:**
1. What percent of total body weight is lean tissue.
2. Knowing this, the recommended body weight can be calculated.

F. **Recommended body weight is defined as the body weight at which there seems to be no harm to human health.**

III. ESSENTIAL AND STORAGE FAT

A. Fat in the human body is classified into two types, essential and stored fat.

1. Essential fat is needed for normal physiological functions.
2. Essential fat constitutes about 3% of the total fat in men and 12% in women.
3. Stored fat is in adipose tissue, mostly beneath the skin and around major organs in the body.
4. Stored fat serves three basic functions:
   a. as an insulator to retain body heat
   b. As energy substrate for metabolism
   c. As padding against physical trauma to the body
5. The amount of storage fat does not differ between men and women:
   a. men tend to store fat around the waist
   b. women tend to store fat around the hips and thighs

IV. TECHNIQUES FOR ASSESSING BODY COMPOSITION

A. Body composition can be assessed through several different procedures:

1. hydrostatic or underwater weighing
2. skinfold thickness
3. girth measurements
4. bioelectrical impedance

B. Because these techniques yield slightlydifferent values, the same technique should be used for pre-test and post-test comparisons.

C. Hydrostatic Weighing:

1. is the most accurate technique. Other techniques to determine body composition are validated against hydrostatic weighing.
2. requires time, space, equipment, and must be administered by a well-trained technician.
3. is not feasible when testing a lot of people, each individual assessment can take as long as 30 minutes.
4. being weighed while submerged underwater makes hydrostatic weighing difficult to administer to those with a fear of water.
5. because of the complexity of hydrostatic weighing, most health and fitness programs prefer measurement techniques which correlate quite well with hydrostatic weighing.

D. Skinfold Thickness

1. Assessing body composition using skinfold thickness gives valid and reliable estimates of the percent body of fat.
2. The skinfold test is done with the aid of pressure calipers.

3. Several sites are measured to reflect the total percentage of fat:
    a. triceps, suprailium, and thigh skinfolds for women
    b. chest, abdomen, and thigh for men
4. Training is necessary to obtain accurate measurements.
5. The same technician should take pre- and post-measurements.
6. And measurements should be done at the same time of the day.
7. All measurements should be taken on the right side of the body.

E. **Girth Measurements:**
1. This simple method measures circumferences at various body sites.
2. This technique requires only a standard measuring tape.
3. Good accuracy can be achieved with little practice:
    a. measurements for women include the upper arm, hip, and wrist
    b. measurements for men include the waist and wrist

F. **Bioelectrical Impedance**
1. The bioelectrical impedance technique is simple to administer.
2. It requires costly equipment.
3. A weak (painless) electrical current is run through the body to analyze body composition.
4. The technique is based on the principle that fat tissue is not as good a conductor of an electrical current as is lean tissue.
5. The accuracy of this technique is still questionable.

G. **Waist-to-Hip Ratio:**
1. Scientific evidence suggests that the way people store fat affects the risk for disease.
2. Individuals who tend to store fat in the abdominal (usually men) are at higher risk for heart disease and other circulatory problems.
3. Those who store fat mainly around the hips and thighs (usually women) are less at risk.
4. A waist-to-hip ratio test was designed assess body composition:
    a. The waist measurement is taken at the point of smallest circumference.
    b. The hip measurement is taken at the point of greatest circumference.
5. Men should lose weight if the waist-to-hip ratio is 1.0 or higher.
6. Women need to lose weight if the ratio is .85 or higher.

H. **Body Mass Index:**
1. Another technique is the Body Mass Index (BMI).
2. This index incorporates height and weight to estimate critical fat values at which the risk for disease increases.
3. BMI is calculated by:
    a. multiplying your weight in pounds by 705
    b. dividing this figure by your height in inches
    c. and then dividing by the same height again

4. According to the BMI:
    a. below 20 -- underweight
    b. 22 to 25 -- lowest risk for chronic disease
    c. 25 to 30 -- classified as overweight
    d. above 30 -- obese
5. BMI is a useful tool to screen the general population, but has the some weaknesses as the height/weight charts.

V. COMPUTING RECOMMENDED BODY WEIGHT

A. After finding percent body fat, body composition can be determined using Table 6.8.

B. In this table you will find the health fitness and the high physical fitness percent fat standards.

1. The health fitness standard is established at the point at which there seems to be no harm to health in terms of percent body fat.
2. A high physical fitness range for women would be between 18% and 23%.
3. The 3% essential fat for men and 12% for women seem to be the lower limits for people to maintain good health. Below these percentages normal physiologic functions can be seriously impaired.

VI. IMPORTANCE OF REGULAR BODY COMPOSITION ASSESSMENT

A. Although most children are not overweight, and most are not overweight when they reach age 20, but starting at age 25 the average man and woman in the U. S. gains 1 pound of weight per year.

B. By age 65, the average American will have gained 40 pounds of weight.

C. Each year the average person also loses a half a pound of lean tissue.

D. Therefore, over this span of 40 years there has been an actual fat gain of 60 pounds accompanied by a 20-pound loss of lean body mass.

E. These changes cannot be detected unless body composition is assessed periodically.

F. If you are on a diet/exercise program, you should repeat your percent body fat assessment and recommended weight computations about once a month.

G. To make valid comparisons, the same technique should be used between pre- and post-assessments.

Instructor Activities

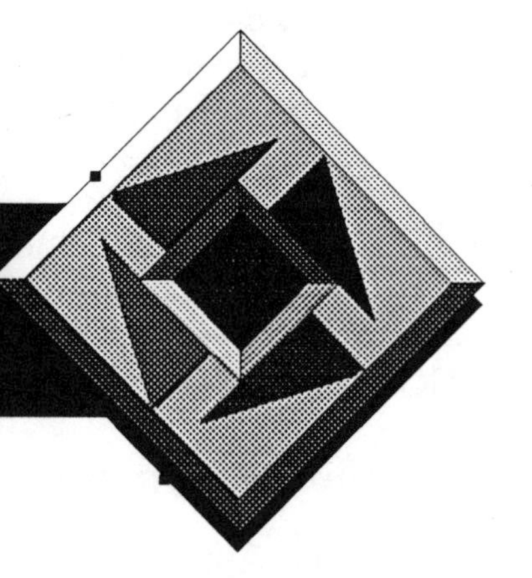

1. **Discuss** the distinction between the fat mass and non-fat or lean body mass components of the body.

2. **Discuss** how medical and health fitness authorities are moving form height/weight charts to body composition in wellness assessments.

3. **Write on the chalkboard,** Total fat, essential fat, and storage fat. Explain the purpose of essential fat and storage fat. Note the difference between males and females.

4. **Show overhead transparency** 36 (in the color transparency packet) or 6-3 (in this manual) to show body compositions according to percent body fat. Note differences in men and women and differences in age.

5. **Show overhead transparency** 15 and 16 (in the color transparency packet) to show how exercise programs can change body composition.

6. **Show overhead transparencies 6-1 and 6.2** (master in this manual) or use the chalkboard to list the various ways of assessing body composition: hydrostatic weighing, skinfold thickness, girth measurements, bioelectrical impedance, waste-to-hip ratio, body mass index. Then compare the techniques in terms of cost, time, ease in administration, accuracy, and purpose.

7. **Demonstrate** the various techniques for assessing body composition. Use overhead transparencies 31, 32, 33 (in the color transparency packet) to show how the tables and figures in the text can be used.

8. **Conduct the assessments** on each student using the technique selected for the class. After finding the percent body fat, have each student determine his or her own body composition classification using the table text or color overhead transparency 36.

TECHNIQUES OF ASSESSING
BODY COMPOSITION

Skinfold Thickness

Men		**Women**
Chest	______	Triceps
+ Abdomen	______	+ Suprailium
+ Thigh	______	+ Thigh
	= ______	...... [see tables]

Girth Measurements

Men *[see table 9.5]*

Waist .... *waist* ______

Wrist .... - wrist ______

= x ______

body weight = y ______

% body fat = x & y on table ______

Women *[find constant for each on table 9.4]*

Upper Arm .... A ______

Age .... - B ______

Hip .... - C ______

Wrist .... + D ______

BD (Body Density) .... = ______

% Body Fat = (495 ÷ BD) - 450 = ______

6-1

TECHNIQUES OF ASSESSING
BODY COMPOSITION

Waste-To-Hip Ratio

Waste (inches) . . . . ______
Hip (inches) . . . . ______
Ratio (waste ÷ hip) . . . . ______
Disease Risk (see Table 9.6) ______

Body Mass Index

Weight (pounds) . . . . ______
Height (inches) . . . . ______
BMI = Weight x 705 ÷ Height ÷ Height
BMI = _____ x 705 ÷ _____ ÷ _____ = ______
Disease Risk (see Table 9.7: ____________________

BMI	Disease Risk
< 20.00	Moderate to Very High
20 to 21.99	Low
22 to 24.99	Very Low
25 to 29.99	Low
30 to 34.99	Moderate
35 to 39.99	High
> 40.00	Very High

6-2

Body CompositionClassification
Accordingto Percent Body Fat

MEN					
Age	Excellent	Good	Moderate	Overweight	Obese
< 19	12.0	12.1-17.0	17.1-22.0	22.1-22.0	>27.1
20-29	13.0	13.1-18.0	18.1-23.0	23.1-28.0	>28.1
30-39	14.0	14.1-19.0	19.1-24.0	24.1-29.0	>29.1
40-49	15.0	15.1-20.0	20.1-25.0	25.1-30.0	>30.1
> 50	16.0	16.1-21.5	21.1-26.0	26.1-31.0	>31.1

WOMEN					
Age	Excellent	Good	Moderate	Overweight	Obese
< 19	17.0	17.1-17.0	22.1-22.0	27.1-32.0	>32.1
20-29	18.0	18.1-23.0	23.1-28.0	28.1-33.0	>33.1
30-39	19.0	19.1-24.0	24.1-29.0	29.1-34.0	>34.1
40-49	20.0	20.1-25.0	25.1-30.0	30.1-35.0	>35.1
> 50	21.0	21.1-26.5	26.1-31.0	31.1-36.0	>36.1

6-3

THE IMPORTANCEOF
REGULAR BODY COMPOSITION ASSESSMENT

- Most children are not overweight, most people 20 are not overweight, but by age 65, the average American is 40 pounds overweight.
- Starting at age 25 the average man and woman in the U. S. gains 1 pound of weight per year.
- Each year the average person also loses a half a pound of lean tissue.
- Therefore, over this span of 40 years there has been an actual fat gain of 60 pounds accompanied by a 20-pound loss of lean body mass.
- These changes cannot be detected unless body composition is assessed periodically.
- Therefore you should repeat your percent body fat assessment and weight computations about once a month.

6-4

Principles of Nutrition for Wellness

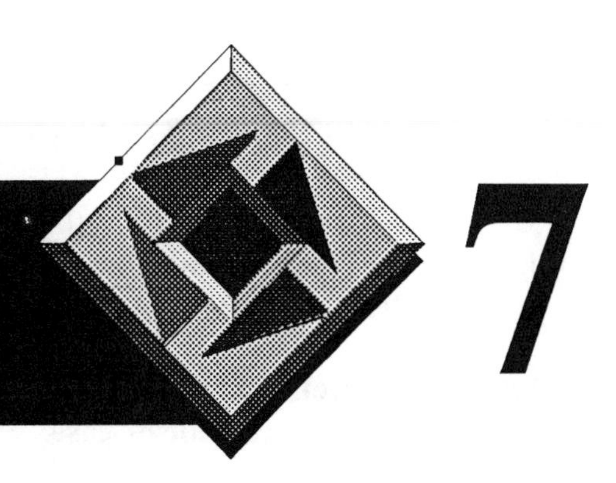

7

Expanded Chapter Outline

I. NUTRITION

A. The science of nutrition studies the relationship of foods to optimal health and performance:

1. Proper nutrition means that a person's diet supplies all the essential nutrients to carry out normal tissue growth, repair, and maintenance.
2. The diet also should provide enough substrates to produce the energy necessary for work, physical activity, and relaxation.
3. These nutrients should be obtained from a wide variety of sources.
4. Too much or too little of any nutrient can precipitate serious health problems.

B. The typical American diet has almost no deficiencies, over consumption is a common problem:

1. is too high in calories, sugar, fat, saturated fat, and sodium
2. is not high enough in fiber
3. these factors undermine good health

C. A 1988 Surgeon General report indicated that diseases of dietary excess and imbalance are among the leading causes of death in the country.

1. Of the total 2.1 million deaths in 1987, an estimated 1.5 million were associated with faulty nutrition.
2. The report said dietary changes can bring better health to all Americans.

D. Nutrition often plays a crucial role in the development and progression of chronic diseases.

1. A diet high in saturated fat and cholesterol increases the risk for atherosclerosis and coronary heart disease.

2. In sodium-sensitive individuals, high salt intake has been linked to high blood pressure.
3. Some researchers believe that 30% to 50% of all cancers are diet-related.
4. Obesity, diabetes mellitus, and osteoporosis also have been associated with faulty nutrition.

E. An effective wellness program must incorporate current dietary recommendations to lower the risk for chronic disease.

F. A summary of guidelines for a healthful diet include:
1. eating a variety of foods
2. avoiding too much fat, saturated fat, and cholesterol
3. eating foods with adequate starch and fiber
4. avoiding too much sugar and sodium
5. maintaining adequate calcium intake
6. maintaining recommended body weight
7. drinking alcoholic beverages in moderation, if at all

II. NUTRIENTS

A. The essential nutrients the human body requires are carbohydrates, fat, protein, vitamins, minerals, and water:
1. Carbohydrates, fat, protein are called fuel nutrients because they supply the energy (calories) needed for work.
2. Vitamins, minerals, and water have no caloric value but still are necessary for a person to function normally and maintain good health.
3. Many nutritionists add fiber to this list of nutrients.
4. Carbohydrates, fats, proteins, and water are termed macronutrients because proportionately large amounts are needed daily.
5. Vitamins and minerals are referred to as micronutrients because the body requires only in small amounts.

B. Foods can be classified as high or low nutrient density depending on the amount of nutrients and calories:
1. High nutrient density refers to foods that contain few or moderate calories but are packed with nutrients.
2. Foods that have a lot of calories but few nutrients are of low nutrient density and commonly are called "junk food."

C. Calorie is the unit of measure indicating the energy value of food and the cost of physical activity.
1. A kilocalorie (kcal) or large calorie is the amount of heat necessary to raise the temperature of 1 kilogram of water one degree Centigrade.
2. People commonly call it a calorie rather than kcal.

III. CARBOHYDRATES

A. Carbohydrates constitute the major source of calories the body uses to provide energy for work, maintain cells, and generate heat:

1. Each gram provides the human body with four calories.
2. The major sources are breads, cereals, fruits, vegetables, and milk and other dairy products.
3. Are classified into simple carbohydrates and complex carbohydrates.

B. Simple Carbohydrates (SUGARS)

1. Monosaccharides:
   a. The simplest sugars, monosaccharides are formed by five- or six-carbon skeletons such as glucose, fructose, and galactose.
   b. Glucose is a natural sugar found in food, but it also is produced in the body from other simple and complex carbohydrates.
   c. Fructose, or fruit sugar, occurs naturally in fruits and honey.
   d. Galactose is produced from milk sugar in the mammary glands of lactating animals.
   e. Both fructose and galactose are converted readily to glucose in the body.
   f. Glucose is used as a source of energy, or it may be stored in the muscles and liver in the form of glycogen.
   g. Glycogen is a long chain of glucose molecules hooked together.
   h. Excess glucose in the blood is converted to fat and stored in adipose (fat) tissue.
   i. Some of it is eliminated by the kidneys through the urine.

2. Disaccharides:
   a. Formed by the linkage of two monosaccharide units, one of which is glucose.
   b. The three major disaccharides are:
      (1) Sucrose or table sugar (glucose + fructose).
      (2) Lactose (glucose + galactose).
      (3) Maltose (glucose + glucose).

C. Complex Carbohydrates

1. Complex carbohydrates or polysaccharides are formed when three or more simple sugar molecules bind together.
2. Complex carbohydrates are starches, dextrins, and glycogen.
   a. Starch is the storage form of glucose in plants.
      (1) Grains, the richest source of starch, should supply most of the energy in a healthful diet.
      (2) Other sources of starch are seeds, corn, nuts, roots, potatoes, and legumes.
      (3) Once eaten, starch is converted to glucose.

b. Dextrins are formed from the breakdown of large starch molecules exposed to dry heat.
   (1) Examples are bread and cold cereals.
   (2) They provide many valuable nutrients and can be an excellent source of fiber.

c. Glycogen is found only in slight amounts in meats.
   (1) Glycogen constitutes the body's reservoirs of glucose.
   (2) Many glucose molecules are linked together to be stored as glycogen in liver and muscle.
   (3) When a surge of energy is needed, enzymes in the muscle break down glycogen into glucose for energy.

IV. DIETARY FIBER

A. Dietary fiber is a type of complex carbohydrate made up of plant material the human body cannot digest.

B. Fiber is important in the diet because it binds water and allows food residues to pass through the intestinal tract more quickly.

C. It is present mainly in leaves, skins, roots, and seeds.

D. Processing and refining foods removes almost all of the natural fiber.

E. In our daily diets the main sources of dietary fiber are whole-grain cereals and breads, fruits, and vegetables.

F. The most common types of fiber are:
1. Cellulose and hemicellulose, found in plant cell walls.
2. Pectins, found in fruits.
3. Gums, also found in small amounts in foods of plant origin.

G. Fiber is either water-soluble or water-insoluble.
1. Pectins and gums are water-soluble fibers.
2. Cellulose and hemicellulose are water-insoluble fibers.

H. Fiber binds water, causing a softer and bulkier stool that increases peristalsis.
1. This moves food residues through the intestinal tract more quickly.
2. Many researchers believe this lowers the risk for colon cancer, because cancer-causing agents are not in contact as long with the intestinal wall.
3. Fiber also is thought to bind with carcinogens and water to lessening the cancer-causing agent's potency.
4. Increased fiber intake also may lower the risk for coronary heart disease because:
   a. fiber may take the place of saturated fats in the diet

b. water-soluble fibers seem to bind cholesterol in the intestines, preventing its absorption

5. Other health disorders, including constipation, diverticulitis, and hemorrhoids have been linked to low fiber intake.

I. The amount of fiber in your diet can be measured either as crude fiber or as dietary fiber.

1. Crude fiber is the smaller portion of the dietary fiber, which actually remains after chemical extraction in the digestive tract.
2. The recommended amount of dietary fiber, 20 to 35 grams per day, contains approximately 7 grams of crude fiber.
3. Most nutrition labels list the fiber content in terms of dietary fiber.

J. Too much fiber in the diet can be detrimental to health.

1. It can produce loss of calcium, phosphorus, and iron.
2. It can also cause gastrointestinal discomfort.
3. When eating more fiber, a person also should drink more water, as too little fluid can cause constipation and even dehydration.

V. FAT

A. There is a distinction between dietary fats which we eat and body fat or adipose tissue.

1. Dietary fat or lipids are used by the human body as a source of energy:
   a. They are the most concentrated energy source.
   b. Each gram of fat supplies nine calories.
2. In addition to providing energy, dietary fat also:
   a. Supplies the body with essential fatty acids
   b. Carries the fat-soluble vitamins A, D, E, and K.
3. Body fat is adipose tissue which stores energy as fat molecules.
   a. Body fat serves as an insulator to preserve body heat.
   b. Body fat also pads the body and absorbs shock.
   c. Fats are also a part of the cell structure.

B. The basic sources of fat are milk and other dairy products, and meats and alternatives.

C. Fats can be classified into three main groups: simple, compound, and derived.

1. Simple Fats:
   a. A simple fat consists of a glyceride molecule linked to one, two, or three units of fatty acids.
      (1) monoglycerides (one fatty acid)
      (2) diglycerides (two fatty acids)
      (3) triglycerides (three fatty acids)
   b. Most of the weight of fat in foods and stored fat in the body are in the form of triglycerides.
   c. Fatty acids are said to be saturated, monounsaturated, or polyunsaturated:

(1) In saturated fatty acids the carbon atoms are fully saturated with hydrogens and only a single bond links the carbon atoms on the chain.
(2) In monounsaturated fatty acids (MUFA) only one double bond is found along the chain.
(3) Polyunsaturated fatty acids (PUFA) contain two or more double bonds between unsaturated carbon atoms along the chain.

d. Saturated fatty acids are mainly of animal origin and unsaturated fats and are found mostly in plant products.
(1) Examples of foods high in saturated fatty acids are meats, meat fat, lard, whole milk, cream, butter, cheese, ice cream, hydrogenated oils, coconut oil, and palm oils.
(2) hydrogenated oils have undergone a process that adds hydrogen to extend shelf-life to keep the oil from separating. Margarine is an example of a transfatty acid.
(3) coconut and palm oils are exceptions to the rule that vegetable oils are unsaturated.
(4) Olive, canola, rapeseed, peanut, and sesame oils, and avocado are examples of monounsaturated fatty acids.
(5) Corn, cottonseed, safflower, walnut, sunflower, and soybean oils are high in polyunsaturated fatty acids.

e. Shorter fatty acid chains also tend to be liquid at room temperature.

f. In general, saturated fats raise the blood cholesterol level, whereas polyunsaturated and monounsaturated fats tend to lower blood cholesterol.

g. Omega-3 fatty acids found in fish seem to be effective in lowering blood cholesterol and triglycerides.
(1) Limited data suggest that eating one or two servings of fish weekly lessens the risk for coronary heart disease.
(2) People with diabetes, a history of hemorrhaging or strokes, on a therapy of aspirin for blood-thinning, and presurgical patients should not consume fish oil except under the physician's instruction.

2. Compound Fats

a. Compound fats are a combination of simple fats and other chemicals. Examples are:
(1) Phospholipids
(2) Glucolipids
(3) Lipoproteins

b. Because lipids do not dissolve in water, lipoproteins transport fats in the blood.

c. Lipoproteins are a combination of lipids covered by proteins.

d. The major forms of lipoproteins are:
(1) high density (HDL)
(2) low density (LDL)
(3) very low density (VLDL) lipoproteins

e. Lipoproteins play a large role in developing or in preventing heart disease:

(1) High HDL (half protein) levels have been associated with a lower risk for coronary heart disease.
(2) High LDL (a fourth protein and half cholesterol) levels have been linked to increased risk for coronary heart disease.
(3) VLDL contains mostly (about half) triglycerides and only about 10% protein and 20% cholesterol.

3. Derived Fats
   a. Derived fats combine simple and compound fats. Sterols, for example, contain no fatty acids. They are considered fats because they do not dissolve in water.
   b. The most often mentioned sterol is cholesterol.
      (1) Cholesterol is found in many foods.
      (2) Cholesterol is also manufactured from saturated fats in the body.

VI. PROTEINS

A. Proteins are the main substances the body uses to build and repair tissues such as muscles, blood, internal organs, skin, hair, nails, and bones..

B. Proteins are a part of the structure of hormones, antibodies which play a key role in all of the body's processes.

C. Proteins can be used as a source of energy, each gram of protein yields four calories of energy.
1. Proteins are used for energy if carbohydrates are not available.
2. Excess proteins may be converted to glucose or fat to be used for energy or stored as fat.

D. The main sources of protein are meats and alternatives, and milk and other dairy products.

E. Proteins are made of amino acids:
1. Humans need about 20 amino acids.
2. Eleven can be manufactured by the body itself.
3. Nine, called essential amino acids, must be obtained from the foods we eat.
4. A complete protein contains all nine essential amino acids.
5. An incomplete protein contains only some of the essential amino acids.
6. An incomplete protein source can be converted to a complete protein if it is combined with a food containing missing essential amino acids.
7. Protein deficiency is not a problem in the usual American diet.
   a. Most Americans eat far too much protein. Only about 12% of your total calories for the day should come from protein.
   b. Two glasses of skim milk combined with about 4 ounces of poultry or fish meet the daily protein requirement.
8. Excess protein can contribute to serious health problems.

a. Proteins from animal sources often are high in fat, saturated fat, and cholesterol, which can lead to cardiovascular disease.
b. Too much animal protein also decreases blood enzymes that prevent precancerous cells from developing into tumors.

9. Protein deficiency, however, could be a concern in some vegetarian diets. The four basic types of vegetarians are:
   a. Vegans, who eat no animal products at all. (Strict vegans also need a supplement of vitamin B12 which is not found in plant foods.)
   b. Ovovegetarians, who allow eggs in the diet.
   c. Lactovegetarians, who eat foods from the milk group.
   d. Ovolactovegetarians, who include egg and milk products in the diet.

VII. VITAMINS

A. Vitamins are organic substances necessary for normal bodily metabolism, growth, and development.

B. Vitamins function as coenzymes which regulate the work of the enzymes.

C. Vitamins are classified into two types based on their solubility:
1. fat-soluble vitamins (A, D, E, and K)
2. water-soluble vitamins (B complex and C)

D. In general, the body does not manufacture vitamins, but obtains them through food we eat.

E. A few exceptions, such as A, D, and K, are formed in the body.
1. Vitamin A is produced from beta-carotene, found in foods such as carrots, pumpkin, and sweet potatoes.
2. Ultraviolet light from the sun changes a compound in the skin called 7-dehydrocholesterol into vitamin D.
3. Vitamin K is created in the body by intestinal bacteria.

F. Vitamins C, E, beta-carotene (a precursor to vitamin A), and the mineral selenium serve as antioxidants.
   a. Antioxidants prevent oxygen from combining with other substances that it may damage.
   b. During metabolism oxygen changes carbohydrates and fats into energy.
   c. In this process a small amount of oxygen ends up in an unstable form referred to as oxygen free radicals.
   d. Solar radiation, cigarette smoke, radiation, and other environmental factors also seem to encourage the formation of free radicals.
   e. Free radicals attack and damage proteins and lipids, in particular the cell membrane and DNA.
   f. This damage is thought to play a key role in the development of conditions such as heart disease, cancer, and emphysema.

g. Researchers believe that antioxidants offer protection by absorbing free radicals before they can cause damage.

VIII. MINERALS

A. Minerals are inorganic elements found in the body and in food.

1. Approximately 25 minerals have important roles in body functioning.
2. Minerals are contained in all cells, especially those in bones, nails, teeth.
3. Minerals are crucial in maintaining water balance and the acid-base balance.
4. Minerals are essential components of pigments and enzymes.
5. Minerals regulate muscular and nervous tissue excitability, blood clotting, and normal heart rhythm.

B. The three minerals mentioned most commonly are:

1. calcium,
2. iron,
3. sodium.

C. The specific functions of some of the most important minerals are given in Table 7.5.

IX. WATER

A. Water is the most important nutrient.

1. Approximately 70% of total body weight is water.
2. Water is involved in almost every vital body process:
   a. in digesting and absorbing food
   b. in the circulatory process
   c. in removing waste products
   d. in building and rebuilding cells
   e. in transporting other nutrients

B. Water is contained in almost all foods but primarily in liquid foods, fruits, and vegetables.

C. Besides the natural content in foods, every person should drink about eight glasses of fluids a day.

X. ENERGY (ATP) PRODUCTION

A. The energy derived from food is NOT used directly by the cells, but is transformed into an energy-rich compound called adenosine triphosphate or ATP.

1. The subsequent breakdown of this compound provides the energy used by all energy-requiring processes of the body.
2. ATP must be recycled continually to sustain life and work.

B. ATP can be resynthesized in three ways.

1. Adenosine Triphosphate and Creatine Phosphate (ATP- CP) system.
   a. The body stores small amounts of ATP and creatine phosphate.
   b. In all-out activities the stores are used up in about 10 seconds.
   c. Then ATP is resynthesized from CP, another high-energy phosphate compound.
   d. Once the CP stores are depleted, the person is forced to slow down or rest to allow ATP to form through anaerobic and aerobic pathways.
2. Anaerobic or lactic acid system.
   a. During high-intensity (anaerobic) exercise ATP is replenished from the breakdown of glucose (only) through a series of chemical reactions that do not require oxygen.
   b. In the process, though, lactic acid is produced, which causes muscular fatigue.
   c. The formation of ATP during anaerobic activities is limited to about 3 minutes.
   d. A recovery period then is necessary to allow for the elimination of lactic acid.
3. Aerobic system.
   a. The production of energy during slow-sustained exercise is derived primarily through aerobic metabolism.
   b. Both glucose (carbohydrates) and fatty acids (fat) are used in this process.
   c. Oxygen is required to form ATP, and under steady state exercise conditions lactic acid accumulation is minimal.
   d. The greater a person's capacity to utilize oxygen the greater is the capacity to generate ATP through the aerobic system.

XI. BALANCING THE DIET

A. One of the fundamental ways to have good health and live life to its fullest is through a well-balanced diet.

B. The recommended guidelines state that daily caloric intake should be distributed as follows:

1. about 58% of the total calories from carbohydrates (48% complex carbohydrates and 10% sugar)
2. less than 30% of the total calories from fat (equally divided [10% each] among saturated, monounsaturated, and polyunsaturated fats)
3. about 12% of the total calories from protein (0.8 grams of protein per kilogram [2.2 pounds] of body weight)
4. The diet also must include all of the essential vitamins, minerals, and water

C. The American diet has changed significantlysince 1900.

1. Diets also were much healthier at the turn of the century.
2. Today people eat more fat, fewer carbohydrates, and about the same amount of

protein, totaling fewer calories.

3. However, we weigh more than our grandparents did, an indication that we are not as physically active.

XII. NUTRIENT ANALYSIS

A. The first step in evaluating your diet is to conduct a nutrient analysis.

1. The analysis covers calories, carbohydrates, fats, cholesterol, and sodium, as well as eight crucial nutrients: protein, calcium, iron, vitamin A, thiamin, riboflavin, niacin, and vitamin C.
2. If the diet has enough of these eight nutrients, the foods consumed typically contain all the other nutrients the human body needs.
3. To do the nutrient analysis, keep a 3-day record of everything you eat.
4. Using the forms in Appendix B, Figure B.1. and the information on the food container to look up the nutrient content for the foods.
5. Total the nutritive values for each day and compute an average for the 3 days.

B. To rate your diet, compare your figures with those in the recommended dietary allowances (RDA) (Table 7.6). This will give you a good indication of:

1. areas of strength
2. areas of deficiency in your current diet.

XIII. ACHIEVING A BALANCED DIET

A. The Healthy Eating Pyramid contained in Figure 7.12 provides simple and sound instructionsfor nutrition.

B. The daily recommended number of servings of the five major food groups are:

1. six to 11 servings of the bread, cereal, rice, and pasta group
2. three to five servings of the vegetable group
3. Two to four servings of the fruit group
4. Two to three servings of the milk, yogurt, and cheese group
5. Two to three servings of the meat, poultry, fish, dry beans, eggs, and nuts group.

C. Phytochemicals is an entirely new field of research with promising results in disease prevention, especially in the fight against cancer.

1. These compounds, just recently discovered by scientists, are found in large quantities in fruits and vegetables.
2. The main function of phytochemicals in plants is to protect them from sunlight.
3. In humans, however, they seem to have a powerful ability to block the formation of cancerous tumors.
4. The recommendation of five to nine servings of fruits and vegetables daily has absolutely no substitute.

D. Milk, poultry, fish, and meats are to be consumed in moderation.

1. Milk should be skim, and milk products should be low-fat.
2. Three ounces of poultry, fish, or meat and not to exceed 6 ounces daily is the recommendation.
3. All visible fat and skin should be trimmed off meats and poultry before cooking.
4. Egg consumption should be limited to no more than three eggs per week.

XIV. NUTRIENT SUPPLEMENTATION

A. According to the Food and Drug Administration:

1. four of every 10 adults in the U. S. take nutrient supplements daily
2. one in every seven has a nutrient intake almost eight times the RDA

B. Most are not needed, vitamin and mineral requirements for the body can be met if the diet contains the recommended servings from the five food groups.

C. People should not take megadoses of vitamins.

1. For most vitamins, a megadose is 10 times the RDA or more.
2. For vitamins A and D, it is respectively five and two times the RDA.
3. Mineral doses should not exceed three times the RDA.

D. Iron supplementation frequently is recommended for:

1. women who have heavy menstrual flow
2. some pregnant and lactating women
3. supplements should be taken under a physician's supervision

E. Other people who may benefit from supplementation are:

1. alcoholics and street-drug users who do not have a balanced diet
2. smokers
3. strict vegetarians
4. individuals on extremely low-calorie diets
5. elderly people who don't eat balanced meals regularly
6. and newborn infants

F. For healthy people with a balanced diet, most supplements do not seem to provide additional benefits. They do not help people:

1. run faster
2. jump higher
3. relieve stress
4. improve sexual prowess
5. cure a common cold
6. boost energy levels

G. Research currently is being done to study the effects of antioxidant supplements, but the effects and amounts of supplements have not been clearly established.

XV. NUTRITION FOR ATHLETES

A. In general, athletes do not require special supplementation or any other special type of diet.

1. Unless the diet is deficient in basic nutrients, no special, secret, or magic diet will help people perform better or develop faster as a result of what they eat.
2. As long as the diet is balanced, based on a large variety of nutrients from the basic food groups, athletes do not require supplements.
3. Even in strength training and body building, protein in excess of 20% of total daily caloric intake is not necessary.
4. The main differences between a sedentary person and a highly active individual is in the total number of calories required.
5. The amount of glycogen is stored in muscle tissue can be increased greatly through carbohydrate loading.
6. A regular diet should be altered during when a person is going to participate in a heavy exercise event of more than 90 minutes.
7. While on a regular diet, the body is able to store between 1,500 and 2,000 calories in the form of glycogen.
8. By following a special diet/exercise regimen 5 days before a long-distance event, highly trained (aerobically) individuals are capable of storing two to three times the amount of glycogen found in the average person.
9. As a rule of thumb, individuals should consume 1 gram of carbohydrate for each 2.2 pounds of body weight 1 hour prior to exercise. The amount of carbohydrate can be increased to 2, 3, or 4 grams per 2.2 pounds of weight 2, 3, or 4 hours, respectively, before exercise.

B. On the day of the long-distance event, high carbohydrates are still the recommended choice. Sugar intake 30 to 45 minutes prior to the event might be counterproductive.

XVI. SPECIAL NUTRITION CONSIDERATIONS FOR WOMEN

A. Women require special nutritional consideration to prevent osteoporosis.

1. Osteoporosis has been defined as the softening, deterioration, or loss of total body bone.
2. The process begins slowly in the third and fourth decades of life.
3. Women are especially susceptible after menopause because of the accompanying estrogen loss.
4. Prevention of osteoporosis begins early in life by having enough calcium in the diet (the RDA is 800 to 1,200 mg per day).
5. A combination of weight-bearing exercises such as walking or jogging and weight training are especially helpful.
6. Current studies indicate that people who are active have denser bone mineral than inactive people do. To have good bone health, people need to participate in a regular lifetime exercise program.

B. Physicallyactive women also may have a greater than average need for iron.

1. Heavy training creates a demand for iron that is higher than the recommended intake.
2. The RDA of iron for adult women is 15 mg per day (10 mg for men).
3. According to a survey by the U.S.D.A., 19- to 50-year-old women consumed only 60% of the RDA for iron.
4. People who do not have enough iron in the body can develop iron deficiency anemia.

XVII. NATIONAL ACADEMY OF SCIENCE'S DIETARY RECOMMENDATIONS

A. The National Academy of Science's Committee on Diet and Health in 1989 issued dietary recommendations for healthy North American adults and children.

B. These guidelines potentially can reduce the risk of developing certain chronic diseases.

1. Reduce fat intake to 30% or less of total calories.
2. Reduce saturated fatty acid intake to less than 10% of total calories and intake of cholesterol to no more than 300 mg daily.
3. Every day eat five or more servings of a combination of vegetables and fruits, especially green and yellow vegetables and citrus fruits.
4. Increase intake of starches and other complex carbohydrates by eating six or more servings daily of a combination of breads, cereals, and legumes.
5. Maintain protein intake at moderate levels (not to exceed 1.6 grams per kilogram of body weight or twice the RDA).
6. Balance food intake and physical activity to maintain appropriate body weight.
7. If you drink alcoholic beverages, limit consumption to the equivalent of less than an ounce of pure alcohol in a single day.
8. Limit total daily intake of salt to 6 grams or less. Limit the use of salt in cooking, and do not add it to food at the table.
9. Maintain adequate calcium intake.
10. Do not take supplements in excess of the RDA in any one day.
11. Maintain an optimal intake of fluoride, particularly during the years of primary and secondary tooth formation and growth.

XVIII. PROPER NUTRITION: A LIFETIME PRESCRIPTION FOR HEALTHY LIVING

A. Proper nutrition, a sound exercise program, and quitting smoking (for those who smoke) are the three factors that do the most for health, longevity, and quality of life.

B. Children tend to eat the way their parents do. If parents adopt a healthy diet, children most likely will follow.

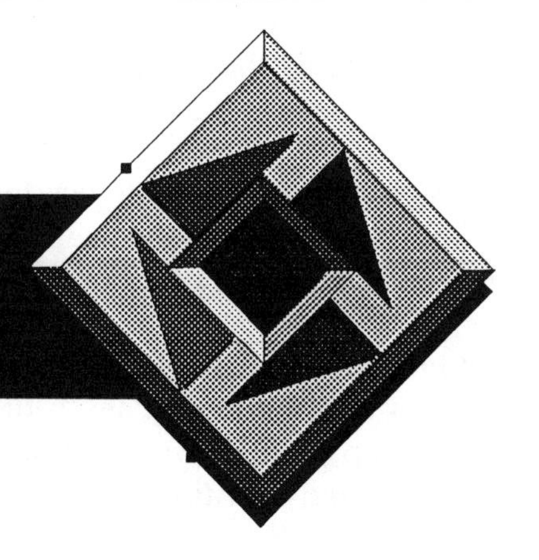

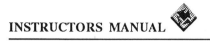

Instructor Activities

1. **Instruct the students** to take a blank sheet of paper and divide it lengthwise into two sections. Ask the students to write the heading, **CURRENT DIET**, at the top of the first column and **DIETARY GOALS** at the top of the second column. Ask them to make notes in the two columns as this lesson continues.

2. **Ask the students** to compare their current eating patterns, the eating patterns in the home where they grew up, and the eating patterns of the typical American family of five decades ago. In which setting is a person most apt to eat better? In years gone by many traditional social and family values were passed on around the dinner table. In today's fast-paced life, perhaps we are missing out on more than proper nutrition.

3. **Ask the students** to discuss other purposes associated with eating besides supplying the body with the nutrients it needs. Eating patterns are sometimes modified by emotions. Business deals are discussed over dinner. Eating is a part of many social activities. These purposes complicate meal planning.

4. **Show overhead transparency 7-1** (from the master in this manual) and discuss the seven elements of nutrition—proteins, fats, carbohydrates, vitamins, minerals, water, and fiber. Discuss the points in the expanded chapter outline. Transparencies 39 and 40 (in the Color Transparency Packet) show specific information about vitamins and minerals.

5. **Use overhead transparencies 41, 47, 37, and 38** (in the color transparency packet) to discuss the relative values of proteins, carbohydrates, and fats as sources of energy. Discuss the types of carbohydrates. Point out the significance of saturated fats and cholesterol in the diet.

6. **Show overhead transparency 7-2,** (from this manual) amd discuss the role of adenosine triphosphate (ATP) or the phosphagen system as it relates to anaerobic and aerobic training. See text page 190 and the expanded outline Section VIII.

6. **Use overhead transparencies 43, 44, and 45** (in the color transparency packet) to discuss the

principles associated with the Food Guide Pyramid. Also use the three dimensional model produced by the Center for Science in the Public Interest displayed on pages 196-7 of the text.

7. **Use overhead transparency 46** (in the color transparency packet) and discuss the information that is avaliable on the new food labels and discuss how this information can be used in planning nutrition for wellness.

8. **Show overhead transparencies 49 and 50** (in the color transparency packet) and discuss the latest information on antioxidants and oxygen-free radicals. Point out that the media often plays up preliminary nutritional research findings. Discuss the problems associated with food fadism and nutritional quackery.

9. **Discuss** the steps a person can take to plan their diet. Use color transparencies 42, 48, and 51 and other charts in this chapter as examples of sources of nutritional information that can be used in tabulating nutrient values. Point out that computer programs are avaliable for personal use in making these tabulations.

THE BASIC NUTRIENTS

PROTEINS	CARBOHYDRATES	FATS
22 amino acids (8 essential) 50 mg. expensive energy → **Structure** **Regulation**	sugar starch complex carbohydrates 1200 cal. ♀ 1500 cal. ♂ **Fuel**	Fatty Acids 30% of diet saturated unsaturated HDLs LDLs **Body Fat**

MINERALS	VITAMINS	WATER	FIBER
macro: calcium, phosphorus, magnesium, potassium, sodium, chloride, sulfur trace: iron, zinc, iodine, copper, fluoride, selenium, chromium, manganese, molybdenum **Structure** **Regulation**	RDA--foods 50-150% – pills fat soluble A D E K water soluble C Ascorbic Acid B1 Thiamin B2 Riboflavin B3 Niacin B6 Pyridoxine B12 Cobalamin Pantothyenuc acid Folacin Biotin **Regulation**	6-8 glasses 60% of body, most critical nutrient **Digestion** **Absorption** **Circulation** **Excretion** **Transportation** **Temperature**	20 grams soluble fruits vegetables cereals legumes whole grains **Intestinal Regularity**

9-1
7-1

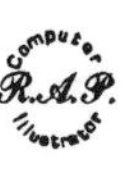

ENERGY IS USED IN ALL BODY PROCESSES

adenosine triphosphate (ATP) or phosphagen system

Energy in Glucose → ATP

Your body uses energy from ATP in all of its processes
Your body stores only small amounts of ATP
(10 to 180 seconds of all-out-activity)
(depending on conditioning)
Then you must rest to allow ATP to be replenished.
There are two systems for replenishing ATP.

Aerobic system.

A chemical reaction when oxygen is available.

slow-sustained exercise
maximum oxygen supply

Glucose + O_2
↓
ATP

(minimal lactic acid accumulation)
The higher the Max VO_2 the greater is the capacity to generate ATP.

7-2

Anaerobic system.

A chemical reactions that does not require oxygen.

high intensity exercise
limited oxygen supply

Glucose (no O_2)
↓ ↓
ATP **lactic acid**

Lactic acid causes muscular fatigue.
Exercise is limited to about 3 minutes.
Then rest is necessary to eliminate lactic acid.

Principles of Weight Control

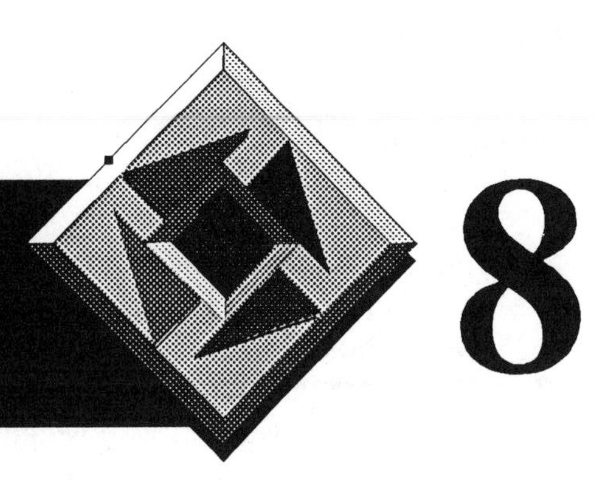

8

Expanded Chapter Outline

I. OBESITY AND OVERWEIGHT

A. In the U.S. about 50% of all women and 25% of all men are on diets.

1. About 65 million are overweight or think they are overweight.
2. Of these, 30 million are obese.
3. People spend about $40 billion yearly attempting to lose weight.

B. Overweight and obesity are not the same thing:

1. Most overweight people are not obese.
2. Obesity applies to the severely overweight.
3. The severely overweight have many health problems.

C. Many people want to lose weight so they will look better:

1. Sometimes they have a distorted image of what is an ideal weight.
2. Only a few have the genes for a "perfect body."
3. People should be realistic as set their own target weight.
4. For many people an excellent percent body fat figure is extremely difficult to attain.
5. It is even more difficult to maintain, unless they are willing to make a lifetime commitment to a dietary and exercise program.
6. Since few people are willing to do that, a moderate percent body fat category may be more realistic:
   a. Ask yourself, Are you happy with your weight?
   b. Part of enjoying a quality of life is being happy with yourself.
   c. If you are not, you should either do something about it or learn to live with it.

D. Many people should lose weight for health reasons.

1. If you are above the moderate category, for health reasons you should try to come down and stay in this category.
2. Being moderately overweight seems to be no detriment to health unless you have another health peoblem such as diabetes or cardiovascular risk factors, then you would benefit from weight loss.
3. If you are in the moderate category ask yoursel:
   a. Do you want to lose weight?
   b. How badly do I want lose it?
   c. Do you want it enough to implement lifetime changes?
   d. If you are not willing to change, you should stop worrying about your weight and deem the moderate category as tolerable.

II. THE WEIGHT LOSS DILEMMA

A. Constantly gaining and losing weight (yo-yo dieting) carries as much health risk as being overweight and remaining overweight.

1. Frequent fluctuations in weight markedly increase the risk of dying from cardiovascular disease.
2. Quick-fix diets should be replaced by a slow but permanent weight loss program.
3. Unfortunately, only about 10% of all people who begin a weight loss program, without exercise, are able to lose the desired weight.
4. Worse, only one in 200 is able to keep the weight off.
5. The body is highly resistant to permanent weight changes through caloric restrictions alone.

B. The $40 billion diet industry tries to capitalize on the idea that weight can be lost quickly.

1. The industry fails to acknowledge the consequences of fast weight loss.
2. The industry fails to consider the importance of lifetime behavioral changes to ensure proper weight loss and maintenance.

C. Various studies indicate most people tend to:

1. underestimate their energy intake
2. overestimate their amount of daily physical activity.
3. Failing to lose weight may be related to misreports of actual food intake and level of physical activity.

D. Fad diets continue to appeal to people with deceptive claim.

1. Most fad diets are low in calories and deprive the body of certain nutrients, generating a metabolic imbalance.
2. With these diets, a lot of the weight lost is in the form of water and protein, and not fat.
3. On a crash diet close to half the weight loss is in lean (protein) tissue.

a. When the body uses protein instead of a combination of fats and carbohydrates as a source of energy, weight is lost faster.
b. Each pound of muscle yields only one-tenth the amount of energy of a pound of fat.
c. As a result, most of the weight loss is in the form of water.

4. Some diets allow only certain specialized foods:
   a. No magic foods provide all of the necessary nutrients, a person has to eat a variety of foods to be well-nourished.
   b. Most of these diets create a nutritional deficiency, which at times can be fatal.
   c. If people realized this, the diet industry would not be as successful.
   d. The reason some of these diets succeed is that people eventually get tired of eating the same thing day in and day out and start eating less.
   e. When they achieve lower weight they start eating normal food again and quickly regain the weight.
5. A few diets do recommend exercise along with caloric restrictions.
   a. The weight loss may be because of the exercise, but the "diet" gets the credit.
   b. If the people do not change their food selection, when they discontinue exercising they gain back the weight quickly.

III. EATING DISORDERS

A. Anorexia nervosa and bulimia are physical and emotional problems, thought to develop from intense fear of becoming fat.

1. Eating disorders involve individual, family, or social pressures.
2. These problems do not disappear even after extreme weight loss.
3. These disorders are increasing steadily in most industrialized nations where society encourages low-calorie diets and thinness.

B. Anorexia Nervosa

1. Anorexia nervosa is a condition of self-imposed starvation.
2. Approximately 19 of every 20 anorexics are young women.
3. About 1% of the female population in the United States is anorexic.
4. Anorexic individuals seem to fear weight gain more than death.
5. They have a distorted image of their body and think of themselves as being fat even when they are emaciated.
6. To speed up the weight loss, they frequently combine extreme dieting, exhaustive exercise, and overuse of laxatives and diuretics.
7. Anorexics commonly develop obsessive and compulsive behaviors and emphatically deny their condition.
8. They are preoccupied with food, meal planning, grocery shopping, and unusual eating habits.
9. As they lose weight and their health begins to deteriorate, they feel weak and tired, but refuse to consider the behavior as abnormal.

10. Malnutrition sets in, physical changes become more visible:
    a. amenorrhea (stopping menstruation), digestive problems
    b. extreme sensitivity to cold
    c. hair and skin problems
    d. fluid and electrolyte abnormalities (irregular heart beat)
    e. injuries to nerves and tendons
    f. abnormalities of immune function
    g. anemia
    h. growth of fine body hair
    i. mental confusion, lethargy, and depression
    j. skin dryness
    k. lower skin and body temperature
11. Many of the changes can be reversed.
12. Treatment almost always requires professional help:
    a. the sooner it is started, the better are the chances for reversibility and cure.
    b. therapy consists of a combination of medical and psychological techniques.
    c. therapy attempts to restore proper nutrition, prevent medical complications, and modify the conditions that triggered the syndrome.
13. Seldom are anorexics able to overcome the problem by themselves.
    a. They strongly deny their condition.
    b. They are able to hide it and deceive their friends and relatives quite effectively.
    c. Anorexia nervosa goes undetected because thinness, dieting, and exercising are socially acceptable.
    d. Only a well-trained clinician is able to make a positive diagnosis.

C. **Bulimia**

1. A pattern of binge eating and purging, bulimia is more prevalent than anorexia nervosa.
    a. For many years it was thought to be a variant of anorexia nervosa, but now it is identified as a separate condition.
    b. It afflicts mainly young people:
        (1) as many as one in five college women
        (2) It also is more prevalent than anorexia nervosa in males
    c. Bulimics usually are healthy-looking people near recommended body weight.
    d. They enjoy food and often socialize around it.
    e. In actuality, they are emotionally insecure and lack self-confidence.
2. The binge-purge cycle usually occurs in stages:
    a. Bulimics anticipate and plan the cycle.
    b. Next they feel an urgency to begin eating.
    c. They feel an uncontrollable urge to consume food.
    d. They experience a short period of relief and satisfaction.
    e. Next they feel guilt, shame, and fear of weight gaining weight.
    f. Purging seems to be an easy answer ao the binging cycle can. continue without fear of gaining weight.

    g. The cycle of binging and purging may last for hours.
3. Bulimics periodically engage in binge eating as a result of stressful life events and a simple compulsion to eat.
4. The most common form of purging is self-induced vomiting.
5. Bulimics frequently ingest strong laxatives and emetics.
6. Medical problems associated with bulimia include:
    a. cardiac arrhythmias
    b. amenorrhea
    c. kidney and bladder damage
    d. ulcers
    e. colitis
    f. tearing of the esophagus or stomach
    g. tooth erosion and gum damage
    h. general muscular weakness
7. Unlike anorexics, bulimics realize their behavior is abnormal and feel great shame about it.
8. Bulimia can be treated successfully when the person realizes this destructive behavior is not the solution to life's problems.
9. A change in attitude can prevent permanent damage or death.
10. Treatment is available on most school campuses through the school's counseling center or the health center.
11. Local hospitals also offer treatment for these conditions.
12. Many communities have support groups, frequently led by professional personnel and usually free of charge.

IV. PHYSIOLOGY OF WEIGHT LOSS

A. Only a few years ago the principles of weight control seemed fairly clear, but we now know the final answers are not in yet.

B. Traditional concepts related to weight control have centered on three points:
1. balancing food intake against energy output
2 that all fat people just eat too much
3. that the human body doesn't care how much fat it stores

C. Although these statements have some truth, they are still open to much debate and research.

D. The Energy-Balancing Equation basically states that:
1. if caloric input equals caloric output, the person will not change weight.
2. if caloric intake exceeds output, the individual gains weight.
3. when output exceeds input, the person loses weight.

E. This principle is simple, but not always the case:
1. since one pound of fat equals 3,500 calories, decreasing daily intake by 500 calories

should result in a loss of 1 pound of fat in 7 days.
2. however, when caloric input is balanced against caloric output, weight loss does not always come as predicted.
3. two people with similar measured caloric intake and output do not necessarily lose weight at the same rate.

F. Explanation for individual differences:
1. variation in human metabolism is the most common explanation.
2. many experts do not believe that metabolism alone is the answer.
3. other theories may better explain these individual variations.

G. Setpoint Theory:
1. This theory involves a weight-regulating mechanism (WRM).
   a. the hypothalamus regulates the appetite and fat storage.
   b. it has a setpoint mechanism that works like a thermostat.
   c. it maintains a fairly constant body weight.
2. Every person's body fat percentage is established by the setpoint:
   a. Some people have high settings.
   b. Some people have low settings.
3. If energy consumption changes the setpoint senses the change.
   a. If consumption decreases the WRM makes the body conserve energy to maintain the "set" weight.
   b. If consumption increases the WRM makes the body expend energy to maintain the "set" weight.

H. Dieting Makes People Fat!
1. Every person has his or her own body fat percentage (setpoint) that the body attempts to maintain. It is a genetic instinct to survive.
2. To lose weight you might reduces your calorie consumption, but the body makes a metabolic adjustment to maintain its setpoint weight.
   a. Your basal metabolic rate may drop dramatically.
   b. This low metabolic rate may counteracts your effort.
   c. With the lower metabolic rate you may actually gain weight.
   d. So you diet more and omit essential nutrients.
3. Very low-calorie diets lower resting metabolic rate and deprive the body of basic daily nutrients required for normal function.
4. A person should not go on a diet below 1,200 and 1,500 calories for women and men, respectively.

I. Changing the setpoint:
1. The setpoint can be lowered so the body will feel comfortable at a lesser fat percentage.
2. Several factors seem to affect the setpoint directly by lowering the fat thermostat:
   a. aerobic exercise
   b. a diet high in complex carbohydrates

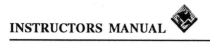

c. nicotine (a distructive alternative)
d. amphetamines (a distructive alternative)
3. On the other hand, several factors seem to raise the setpoint:
a. a diet high in fats and refined carbohydrates
b. near-fasting diets
c. artificial sweeteners (perhaps)
4. The only sensible way to lower the setpoint seems to be a combination of aerobic exercise and a diet high in complex carbohydrates.
5. Many nutritionists believe the source of calories rather than the number of calories should be the concern in a weight-control program.
a. continue to eat the same amount
b. increase the complex carbohydrates and high-fiber foods
c. decrease the refined carbohydrates (sugars) and fats
d. this will decrease total daily caloric intake
6. A "diet" should viewed NOT as a temporary tool, but as a permanent change in eating behaviors.
7. The role of increased physical activity is also immportant.

J. Diet and Metabolism
1. In weight loss by dietary restrictions alone, lean body mass (muscle protein and vital organ protein) always decreases.
2. When obese people go on a near-fasting diet, only half of the weight loss is actually fat, the rest is lean body mass.
3. When the diet is combined with exercise, nearly all of the weight loss is in the form of fat, and lean tissue actually may increase.
4. Loss of lean body mass is never good, it can:
a. weaken muscles
b. damage organs
c. slow down metabolism
d. cause disturbances in heart function
5. Overindulging (binge) followed by very-low-calorie diets is not good:
a. it may change the metabolic rate
b. it may change the electrolyte balance
6. Aging and metabolic rates:
a. aging is not the main reason for lower metabolic rate
b. the metabolic rate slows down because people slow down
c. as people age, we tend to rely more on the amenities of life (remote controls, cellular telephones, single-level homes) that lull us into sedentary living
7. Basal metabolism is related directly to body composition.
a. Metabolism is the proscess of using oxygen to burn calories.
b. The body requires a certain amount of oxygen per pound of lean body mass.
c. Since metabolism provides the oxygen; the more lean tissue, the higher is the metabolic rate.
d. Exercises that build muscles increase the demand for oxygen.
e. Each additional pound of muscle tissue can raise the basal metabolic rate

between 30 and 50 calories per day.
   f. Muscles burn calories 24 hours a day, even when the body is at rest.
   g. With less physical activity, lean mass decreases and fat increases.
   h. Fat is metabolically inert, has no energy requirements.
8. Diets with caloric intakes below 1,200 to 1,500 calories may not allow retention of lean body mass.
9. At this intake level, some loss in lean body mass is inevitable unless the diet is combined with exercise.
10. Despite the claims of many diets, regardless of the nutrients added, severe caloric restrictions prompt a loss of lean tissue.

V. EXERCISE: THE KEY TO WEIGHT LOSS AND WEIGHT MAINTENANCE

A. Based on the preceding discussion, exercise is vital to losing weight and maintaining that weight loss.

B. If a person is trying to lose weight, a combination of aerobic and strength-training exercises works best.

C. If a person is running 3 miles per per day (300 calories burned), three days per week, 13.5 extra pounds of fat will be burned in one year.

D. An individual who adds 5 pounds of muscle tissue can burn the calorie equivalent of 15.6 pounds of fat per year.

VI. HEALTHY WEIGHT GAIN

A. "Skinny" people, too, should realize that the only healthy way to gain weight is through exercise and a slight increase in caloric intake.

B. Attempting to gain weight just by overeating will raise the fat component and not the lean component.

C. A strength training program is the best approach to add body weight.

D. To produce the most muscle hypertrophy, the program should include at least:
1. two exercises for each major body part
2. do three to five sets with about 10 repititions
3. see Principles Involved in Strength Training in Chapter 4.

VII. WEIGHT LOSS MYTHS

A. **Spot reducing:**
1. When fat comes off, it affects the entire body, not just specific areas.
2. The greatest proportion of fat comes off the greatest fat deposits.

B. **Losing "cellulite":**
1. These deposits are nothing but accumulations of enlarged fat cells.
2. A few special exercises will not get rid of fat in a specific part of the body.

C. **Wearing rubberized sweatsuits:**
1. Sweatsuits hasten the rate of body fluid loss.
2. This also raises the core temperature of the body.
3. This combination puts a person in danger of dehydration.

D. **Steam baths or saunas:**
1. Time in a sauna can show a weight loss on the scale immediately afterward,
2. But as soon as you replace body fluids, you gain back the weight.

E. **Mechanical vibrators:**
1. Vibrating belts and rollers may feel good, but they require no effort.
2. Fat cannot be rolled of shaken off, in weight control they are worthless.

VIII. LOSING WEIGHT THE SOUND AND SENSIBLE WAY

A. **People who are overweight and are serious about losing weight have to include regular exercise along with proper food management in a sensible weight reduction program.**

B. **Some precautions are in order, as excessive body fat may be a major risk factor, but unwise weight reduction can also precipitate serious health problems.**

C. **Depending on the extent of the weight problem, a medical examination may be appropriate before undertaking the exercise program.**

D. **A person should not try to do too much too fast.**

IX. TIPS FOR BEHAVIOR MODIFICATION

A. **Modifying old habits and developing new, positive behaviors take time.**

B. **Individuals have successfully applied the following management techniques.**

C. **People might use only the stratigies that apply to them:**
1. Make a commitment to change.

2. Set realistic goals.
3. Incorporate exercise into the program.
4. Develop healthy eating patterns.
5. Avoid automatic eating.
6. Stay busy.
7. Plan your meals ahead of time.
8. Cook wisely.
9. Do not serve more food than you should eat.
10. Eat slowly and at the table only.
11. Avoid social binges.
12. Beware of raids on the refrigerator and the cookie jar.
13. Avoid eating out.
14. Practice stress management techniques.
15. Monitor changes and reward accomplishments.
16. Think positive.

TRIVIA NOTE

What do the numbers stand for?

63, 50, 25, 10, 15, 5, 1, .05, .005

The number **63** is the percent of the adult population of the United States who are over their recommended weight range.Numbers **50** and **25** is the percent of all women and men respectively on diets at any given time. Number **10** is the percent of all people who begin a weight loss program without exercise who reach their goal and **.005** is the percent who keep it off. Number **5** is the percent of college women who may be bulimic and **1** is the percent of all American females who are anorexic. Number **.05** is the percent of anorexics who are male, the number of male balimics is a little higher.

THE COST OF WEIGHT LOSS FRAUD

Point out that dieting myths lead Americans to spend more than $10 billion a year on weight loss. After a year most of the people who spend this money have nothing to show for their investment. In fact most of them are worse off a few months after their diets. They may loose more than their money.

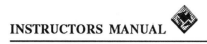

Instructor Activities

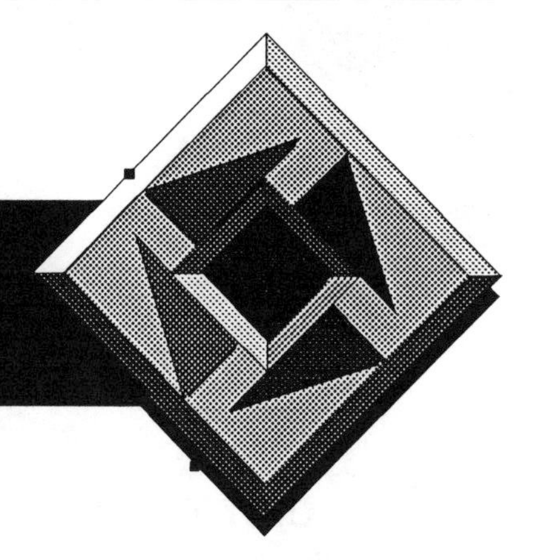

1. **Write on the chalkboard** the numbers in the trivia note on the previous page and ask the students who are trivia buffs what the number stands for.

2. **Show overhead transparency** 8-1 and discuss the dieting myths. The students will be able to add some that are not listed on the transparency or in the text. Also talk about the fallacies surrounding the loss of cellulite, the concept of spot-reducing, the use of rubberized sweatsuits, and mechanical vibrators.

5. **Show overhead transparency** 8-2 and discuss the setpoint theory. Ask, why is it called a theory? What parts of it are facts and what parts are theory?

6. **Use the chalkboard** to show the formula:
   Calories consumed - calories expended = weight gain or loss
   Point out that this formula is essentially true, but it is not that simple. Recent discoveries show that there are many variables affecting weight management and more research will reveal additional information. Although one pound of fat equals 3,500 calories, consuming or expending 3,500 calories will not necessarily result in a pound of fat gained or lost.

7. **Show overhead transparency** 18 (from the Color Transparency Packet) to show the effects of three forms of diet on fat loss (see text page 226 and expanded outline Section V).

8. **Show overhead transparency** 17 (from the Color Transparency Packet) to show the changes in body composition as a result of a combined aerobic and strength training program.

9. **Show overhead transparency** 19 (from the Color Transparency Packet) to show the value of aerobic exercise in weight loss and maintenance.

10. **Show overhead transparencies** 8-3, 8-4, and 8-5 and discuss eating disorders. These are serious problems at most colleges. Perhaps the emphasis on thinness in physical education and health courses over the years has contributed to this problem.

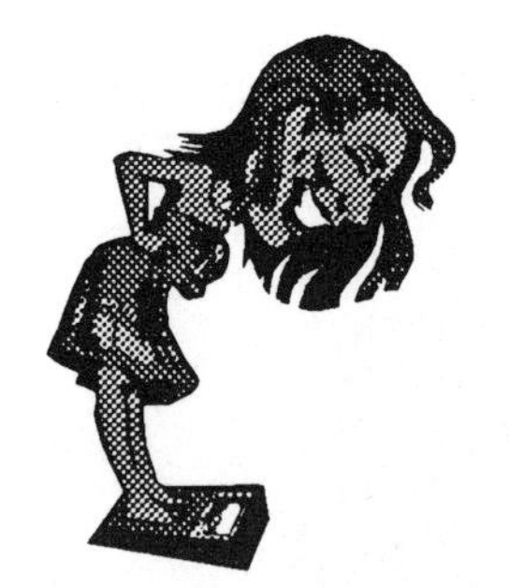

DIETING MYTH

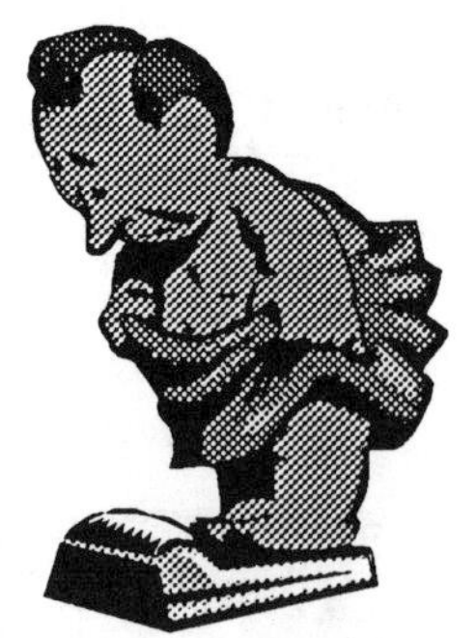

Most diets are myths
because they provide only temporary weight loss.

- The diet calls for **only certain foods**.
  - People get tired of eating the same old thing.
  - So they start eating less and lose weight.
  - When they start eating again they gain back the weight.

- **Crash diets** produce rapid weight loss.
  But the loss is water and protein, not fat.
  - Metabolized muscle protein
    (1/5 energy, 4/5 excreted as water)
  - Most of the weight loss is water.
  - The water and the weight will soon return.

- Most diets **low in calories** are also low in other important nutrients.
  - This deprives the body of certain nutrients.
  - It may cause a metabolic imbalance.

8-1

SETPOINT THEORY

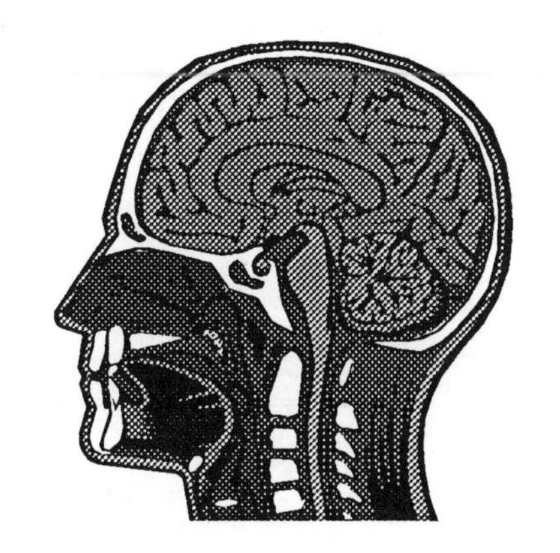

The hypothalamus regulates the appetite and fat storage. It works like a thermostat.

Every person's body fat percentage is established. The setpoint tends to keep weight consistent.

When the diet changes the body makes metabolic adjustments to maintain that percent.

- ▾ When calories are reduced, the metabolic rate may drop to try to prevent weight loss. With a lower metabolic rate the person tends to gain weight. Eating less may promote a weight gain.

- ▾ When calories are increased, the metabolic rate may increase to prevent weight gain. With a higher metabolic rate the person tends to lose weight. Eating more may promote weight loss.

- ▾ Several behaviors have been shown to lower the fat thermostat and increase the metabolic rate.
  - — Aerobic exercise
  - — A diet high in complex carbohydrates
  - — Nicotine and amphetamines (these are more destructive than being overweight).

8-2

ANOREXIA NERVOSA

Anorexia nervosa is
a condition of self-imposed starvation.

1% of all American females are anorexic.
1 of 20 anorexics are male.

BACKGROUND

- They appear to be successful and to get along well with other people.
- They feel uncertain about their identity, their coping skills, and their powers of personal control.
- They are constantly preoccupied with food, and dieting provides a sense of being in control.
- They see themselves as being fat even when they are emaciated.
- They fear weight gain more than death by starvation.
- Their striving for rapid weight loss may combine:
  extreme dieting, exhaustive exercise, and use of laxatives and diuretics.
- They emphatically deny that they have a problem.

8-3

ANOREXIA
MEDICAL PROBLEMS

- ▾ malnutrition
- ▾ amenorrhea (stopping menstruation)
- ▾ digestive problems and anemia
- ▾ extreme sensitivity to cold
- ▾ the skin becomes dry
- ▾ they grow fine body hair
- ▾ electrolyte abnormalities lead to heart problems
- ▾ abnormalities of immune function,
- ▾ mental confusion, lethargy, and depression

DETECTION

- ▾ They strongly deny their condition.
- ▾ They hide it from friends and relatives.
- ▾ Exercising and dieting are socially acceptable.
- ▾ Only clinicians are able to make a diagnosis.

TREATMENT

- ▾ Professional treatment is almost always required.
- ▾ The sooner the treatment is started, the better.
- ▾ Many of the medical problems can be reversed.
- ▾ Therapy combines medical and psychological techniques.

8-4

BULIMIA

Bulimia is a pattern of binge eating and purging.

One in five college women may be bulimic.

- **Physically** bulimics usually look healthy.
- **Emotionally** they are insecure.
- **Socially** they enjoy food and socialize around it.
- Eating and maintaining weight are important.
- Compulsively they binge periodically.
- This is followed by purging—vomiting, emetics, diuretics)

MEDICAL PROBLEMS

- cardiac arrhythmias
- amenorrhea
- kidney and bladder damage
- ulcers, colitis, tearing of the esophagus
- tooth erosion, gum damage

TREATMENT

- Bulimics realize their behavior is abnormal and destructive, they feel shame, and may seek help.

- Bulimia can be treated successfully. If help is obtained in time it can prevent permanent damage.

8-5

Principles of Weight Control

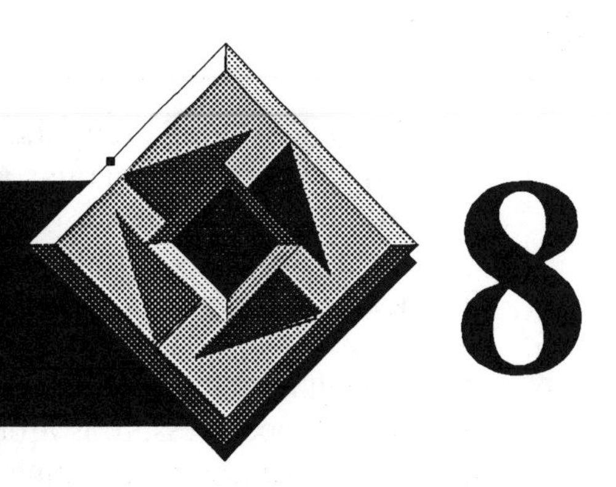

8

Expanded Chapter Outline

I. CARDIOVASCULAR DISEASE

A. Cardiovascular disease is the leading cause of death in the United States:

1. It accounts for nearly half of the total mortality rate.
2. It costs the nation well over $135 billion annually.

B. The disease encompasses any pathological condition that affects the heart and the circulatory system (blood vessels).

1. Some examples of cardiovascular disease are:
    a. coronary heart disease
    b. peripheral vascular disease
    c. congenital heart disease
    d. rheumatic heart disease
    e. stroke
    f. high blood pressure
    g. congestive heart failure
    h. atherosclerosis
2. The major cardiovascular disease is coronary heart disease (CHD), a narrowing of the coronary arteries:
    a. The arteries are blocked by fatty deposits such as cholesterol.
    b. This diminishes the supply of oxygen and nutrients to the heart.
    c. And this can precipitate a heart attack.
3. Almost all of the risk factors for CHD are preventable and reversible:
    a. Genetic inheritance plays a role in CHD.
    b. But the most important determinant is personal lifestyle.
    c. The specific objectives of a CHD risk factor analysis are to:
        (1) screen individuals who may be at high risk.

(2) educate regarding the leading risk factors.
(3) implement programs aimed at reducing the risk.
(4) use the analysis as a starting point from which to compare changes induced by the intervention program.

4. The leading risk factors contributing to CHD are listed in Table 9.1.
5. A self-assessment CHD risk factor analysis is given in Figure 9.3.
6. The guidelines for zero risk are outlined for each factor; for example:
   a. ideal blood pressure is around 120/80 or lower.
   b. risk is reduced by smoking less or quitting altogether.
   c. HDL should be 45 mg/dl or higher for men (55 for women).
   d. LDL should be less than 170 mg/dl.
7. The CHD risk factor-analysis is used to identify risk categories:
   a. "very low" designates the group at lowest risk.
   b. "low" suggests that healthy people can still improve.
   c. "moderate" means the person can definitely improve.
   d. "high" or "very high" points to a strong probability of developing heart disease within the next few years and calls for an immediate personal risk reduction program.

II. LEADING RISK FACTORS

A. The leading risk factors contributing to CHD are:

1. Physical inactivity
2. Low HDL-cholesterol and or Elevated LDL-cholesterol
3. Elevated triglycerides
4. Smoking
5. High blood pressure
6. Abnormal stress or resting electrocardiogram
7. Family history of heart disease (genetic inheritance)
8. Personal history of heart disease
9. Diabetes
10. Excessive body fat
11. Tension and stress
12. Age

B. Most risk factors are preventable and reversible.

C. Multiple interrelations usually exist between risk factors:

1. Physical inactivity is related to body fat, cholesterol, stress, and high blood pressure.
2. Smoking is related high blood pressure.

III. PHYSICAL INACTIVITY

A. The American Heart Association lists four major factors of disease:

1. Physical activity
2. Smoking
3. High blood pressure
4. Abnormal cholesterol

B. Dr. Kenneth H. Cooper, pioneer of the aerobic movement, and many other researchers have found evidence of the benefits of aerobic exercise in reducing heart disease.

C. Improving cardiovascular endurance through aerobic exercise may have the greatest impact in reducing overall risk for heart disease.

1. Aerobic exercise will:
   a. increase cardiovascular endurance
   b. decrease and control blood pressure
   c. reduce body fat
   d. lower blood lipids (cholesterol and triglycerides)
   e. improve HDL-cholesterol
   f. help control diabetes
   g. increase and maintain good heart function
   h. motivate toward smoking cessation
   i. alleviate tension and stress
   j. counteract a personal history of heart disease
2. The basic principles for cardiovascular exercise are given in Chapter 3.

IV. ABNORMAL ELECTROCARDIOGRAM

A. The electrocardiogram (ECG) is a valuable measure of the heart's function:

1. The ECG provides a record of the electrical impulses that stimulate the heart to contract.
2. In reading an ECG, five general areas are interpreted:
   a. heart rate
   b. heart rhythm
   c. axis of the heart
   d. enlargement or hypertrophy of the heart
   e. myocardial infarction or heart attack
3. The EKG provides a "pictures" of the electrical impulses traveling through the heart and can indicate abnormalities in heart functions.
4. A stress EKG should be administered to the following:
   a. men over age 40 and women over age 50
   b. a total cholesterol level above 200 mg/dl or an HDL-cholesterol below 35 mg/dl
   c. hypertensive and diabetic patients
   d. cigarette smokers
   e. individuals with a family history of CHD, syncope, or sudden death before age

60

f. people with an abnormal resting ECG

g. all individuals with symptoms of chest discomfort, dysrhythmia, syncope, or chronotropic heart incompetence

V. ABNORMAL CHOLESTEROL PROFILE

A. Cholesterol is a waxy substance found only in animal fats and oil:

1. It is essential for specific metabolic functions in the body.
2. As a part of the skin it acts as a moisture barrier.

B. An abnormal cholesterol profile contributes to atherosclerotic plaque:

1. A buildup of fatty tissue in the walls of the arteries.
2. Plaque blocks the vessels that supply the heart muscle with oxygen.
3. The obstructions can trigger a myocardial infarction or heart attack.
4. Cholesterol is carried in the bloodstream by molecules of protein.
5. High density lipoprotein (HDLs).
6. Low-density lipoprotein (LDLs).
7. Very low-density lipoprotein (VLDLs).

C. LDLs tend to release cholesterol in transit:

1. Cholesterol tends to penetrate the lining of the arteries.
2. It speeds up the process of atherosclerosis—plaque formation.

D. HDLs do not release cholesterol in transit.

1. They act as *scavengers*, removing cholesterol from blood.
   a. tends to attract cholesterol.
   b. carries it to the liver to be metabolized and excreted.
2. This prevents plaque from forming in the arteries.
3. HDL is the *good cholesterol*, it offers some heart risk protection.
4. The more HDL-cholesterol, the better.

E. Blood tests are used to determine the amount of cholesterol in the blood:

1. A total cholesterol (blood lipid) includes LDLs and LDLs.
2. A differential test lists LDLs and HDLs separately.
3. Values are stated in milligrams of cholesterol per deciliter of blood.

F. National guidelines for cholesterol values state:

1. Total cholesterol:
   a. under 200 mg/dl is desirable.
   b. 200-239 mg/dl is borderline high.
   c. over 240 mg/dl is a high risk.
2. LDL-cholesterol:
   a. below 130 mg/dl is desirable.

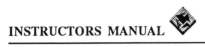

b. 130 and 159 mg/dl is borderline high.
c. over 160 mg/dl is a high risk.

3. HDL-cholesterol:
   a. over 45 mb/dl is desirable.
   b. 36-44 mg/dl is a modest risk.
   c. under 35 mg/dl is a high risk.

G. HDL-cholesterol is determined genetically and generally:

1. Women have higher values than men.
2. Blacks have higher values than caucasians.
3. HDL-cholesterol also decreases with age.

H. Some behaviors tend to increase HDLs:

1. Habitual aerobic exercise
2. Weight loss
3. Quitting smoking
4. Beta-carotene and drug therapy also promote higher HDL levels

I. The relationship between diet and cholesterol is complex:

1. The average adult consumes 400 to 600 mg of cholesterol daily.
2. The liver manufactures another 1000 mg of cholesterol per day.
   a. most of this is produced from saturated fats
   b. there are wide individual differences
      (1) some people consume high amounts of saturated fats and still maintain normal cholesterol levels
      (2) some people with a lower intake can have abnormally high cholesterol levels
3. If LDL-cholesterol is higher than recommended, it can be lowered by:
   a. taking medication
   b. losing body fat
   c. manipulating the diet
      (1) low in fat, saturated fat, and cholesterol (10% of total diet)
      (2) high in complex carbohydrates and fiber
4. To lower LDL-cholesterol levels, the following general dietary guidelines are recommended:
   a. consume fewer than three eggs per week
   b. eat red meats (3 oz. serving) fewer than three times per week
   c. do not eat commercially baked foods
   d. drink low-fat milk (1%) and low-fat dairy products
   e. do not use coconut oil, palm oil, or cocoa butter
   f. eat fish twice a week. (fish high in Omega-3 fatty acids include mackerel, herring, tuna, salmon, and lake trout)
   g. bake, broil, grill, poach, or steam food instead of frying
   h. refrigerate cooked meat (so you can remove the hardened fat) before adding to other dishes

i. avoid fatty sauces made with butter, cream, or cheese
j. maintain recommended body weight

VI. ELEVATED TRIGLYCERIDES

A. Triglycerides in combination with cholesterol speed plaque formation:
1. These fatty acids are carried in the bloodstream by VLDLs.
2. They are found in poultry skin, lunch meats, and shellfish.
3. They are also manufactured in the liver, from sugars and alcohol.
4. They can be lowered by:
   a. cutting down on these foods
   b. reducing weight (if overweight)
   c. doing aerobic exercise

B. An optimal blood triglyceride level is less than 100 mg/dl (see Table 11.2).

C. Some people have a genetic condition which causes elevated triglycerides:
1. 40% of the population has a condition is called LDL phenotype B.
2. Although blood lipids may not be high, they are at higher risk.

D. Everyone should have had a blood chemistry test:
1. An initial test establishes a baseline for future reference.
2. A blood analysis every 3 years prior to age 35.
3. After age 35, individuals should have a blood lipid test every year.

VII. DIABETES

A. In diabetes mellitus the blood glucose is unable to enter the cells:
1. Insulin is a hormone produced in the pancreas.
2. Insulin helps the cells use glucose.
3. In diabetes, insufficient insulin is produced to meet the body's needs:
   a. production may totally stop
   b. production may be insufficient
4. The two major types of diabetes are:
   a. Type I, or insulin-dependent diabetes—juvenile diabetes
   b. Type II, or non-insulin-dependent diabetes—adult-onset
   c. there is a genetic predisposition to diabetes

B. Adult-onset diabetes is related closely to:
1. a genetic predisposition
2. overeating
3. obesity
4. lack of physical activity

C. In most cases this condition can be corrected through:
1. a special diet
2. a weight-loss program
3. a regular exercise program

D. Aerobic exercise seems to helps prevent diabetes due to less body fat and better sugar and fat metabolism.

E. Individualswho have high blood glucose levels should consult a physician to decide on the best treatment.

VIII. HYPERTENSION

A. Blood pressure is a measure of the force exerted against the walls of the blood vessels by the blood flowing through them.

B. Blood pressure is assessed using a sphygmomanometer and a stethoscope:
1. The sphygmomanometer or blood pressure cuff is an inflatable bladder.
2. It has a manometer from which the pressure is read.
3. The reading is equivalent to milliliters of mercury.
4. The reading is expressed in two numbers:
   a. systolic—the higher number—during heart contraction.
   b. diastolic—the lower number—when the heart is relaxed.
5. Ideal blood pressure should be 120/80 or below:
   a. systolic 121 to 139 and/or diastolic 81-89—borderline high.
   b. systolic over 140 and/or diastolic over 90—hypertension.

C. Blood pressure may fluctuate during a regular day:
1. Many factors affect blood pressure—activity, stress, relaxation.
2. A single reading may not be a true indicator of your real pressure.

D. Hypertension has been called the silent killer:
1. It does not hurt, it does not make you feel sick.
2. Unless you check it, you may not realize you have a problem.
3. High blood pressure is also a risk factor for congestive heart failure, strokes, and kidney failure.

E. Hypertension killsby contributingto atherosclerosis.
1. The inner lining of arteries walls are normally smooth.
2. Blood lipids cannot penetrate the lining unless it is damaged.
3. As blood pressure rises it damages the lining of the arteries.
4. The higher the pressure, the greater is the damage.
5. Damaged walls are susceptible to fat deposits called atherosclerosis.
6. Deposits of cholesterol and other fats block the arteries.

7. Blocked arteries reduce the blood supply to the heart and brain.
8. A decreased blood supply can lead to a heart attack or stroke.

F. Constant high blood pressure also causes congestive heart failure.

G. High blood pressure also damages blood vessels to the kidneys, eyes, and other parts of the body.

H. There are two types of hypertension, 90% is essential hypertension and 10% is caused by pathological conditions.

1. Essential hypertension has no definite cause and is treatable with:
   a. aerobic exercise
   b. weight reduction
   c. low sodium/high potassium diet
   d. stress reduction
   e. no smoking
   f. diet to reduce blood lipids
   g. antihypertensive medication
2. Physicians will usually try behavioral changes before medications:
   a. antihypertensive medicines are often prescribed.
   b. but they produce many multiple side effects.
   c. because of the side effects, many patients stop taking the medication.

I. A factor contributing to high blood pressure is too much sodium (salt).

1. Sodium is essential for normal body functions:
   a. the body requires 200 mg, or a tenth of a teaspoon daily.
   b. a typical American gets between 6,000 and 20,000 mg per day.
2. With high sodium intake the body may retains more water.
3. This increases the blood volume and increases blood pressure.

J. The link between hypertension and obesity has been well-established.

1. Blood pressure increase with excess body fat.
2. Capillaries are constricted by the adipose tissues they run through.
3. Every additional pound of fat requires an extra mile of blood vessels.
4. The heart muscle must work harder to pump the blood through a longer, constricted network of blood vessels.

K. Aerobic exercise plays a major role of in managing blood pressure.

1. Cardiovascularly fit individuals have lower blood pressures.
2. Aerobic exercise often is prescribed for hypertensive patients.
3. Exercise, not weight loss, is the main contributor to lowered blood pressure.
4. Exercise programs for hypertensive patients should be of moderate intensity.
5. High-intensity training in hypertensive patients actually may cause the blood pressure to rise slightly.

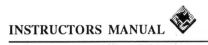

L. Most important is a preventive approach. Keeping blood pressure under control is easier than trying to bring it down once it is high.

1. Regardless of your past blood pressure history, high or low, you should check it routinely.
2. Regular physical exercise, weight control, a low-salt diet, no smoking, and stress management are the keys to controlling blood pressure.

IX. EXCESSIVE BODY FAT

A. Body composition is the ratio of lean body weight to fat weight:

1. If the body contains too much fat, the person is considered obese.
2. Obesity long has been recognized as a primary risk factor for CHD.

B. Too much body fat is a serious coronary risk factor:

1. Attaining recommended body composition is important in decreasing cardiovascular risk.
2. A positive thing about this risk factor is that it can be removed through a combination of diet and exercise.
3. Recommendations for weight management are discussed in Chapter 10.

X. SMOKING

A. Cigarette smoking is the single largest preventable cause of illness and premature death in the United States:

1. Smoking has been linked to:
   a. cardiovascular disease
   b. cancer
   c. bronchitis
   d. emphysema
   e. peptic ulcers

B. In coronary disease:

1. Smoking speeds up the process of atherosclerosis.
2. It also increases the risk of death following a heart attack.

C. Smoking release nicotine into the bloodstream:

1. Nicotine is a vaso-constrictor, it constricts the size of arteries.
2. It constricts the coronary arteries serving the heart muscle.

D. Smoking puts another 1,200 toxic compounds into the bloodstream:

1. Many of these substances damage the lining of the arteries.
2. The damaged linings attract cholesterol and triglycerides.
3. Plaque builds up to obstruct bloodflow through the arteries.
4. Smoking also encourages the formation of blood clots.

5. The clots can completely block an artery narrowed by atherosclerosis.

E. Carbon monoxide is a byproduct of combustion while one is smoking.
1. Carbon monoxide decreases the blood's oxygen-carrying capacity.
2. Obstructed arteries and less oxygen heightens the risk for heart problems.

F. Smoking also:
1. Increases heart rate.
2. Raises blood pressure.
3. Decreases the production of HDL-cholesterol.

G. Smoking presents a greater risk for heart disease than for lung disease:
1. Pipes, cigars, and chewing tobacco increase the risk for heart disease.
2. Toxic substances are absorbed through the membranes of the mouth.

XI. TENSION AND STRESS

A. Tension and stress have become a normal part of life:
1. It is not the stressor, but the response to it, that is the health hazard.
2. The human body responds to stress by producing emergency hormones.
3. These hormones elevate heart rate and blood pressure to prepare for action.
4. Physical activities metabolize the hormones and the body returns to normal.
5. But, if a person is unable to take action the hormones remain elevated.

B. People who are unable to relax put a constant low-level strain on the cardiovascular system that could manifest itself in heart disease:
1. Under stress the coronary arteries constrict.
2. This reduces the oxygen supply to the heart.
3. If the blood vessels are already blocked by atherosclerosis the results may be worse, abnormal heart rhythms or even a heart attack may follow.

C. PERSONAL AND FAMILY HISTORY

D. If you have had cardiovascular problems in the past, your risk is higher:
1. You should try hard to control the other risk factors.
2. Most risk factors are reversible.
3. The more time that has passed since a problem, the lower the risk.

E. Genetic predisposition toward heart disease has been well demonstrated:
1. The risk is higher if blood relatives have had heart disease before age 60.
2. The younger the age, the greater the risk of a genetic predisposition.
3. It is hard to tell if a problem was due to genetics or lifestyle.

F. A person with a family history of cardiovascular problems should watch all other factors

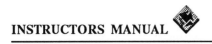

closely and maintain as low a risk level as possible.

XII. AGE

A. **Age is a risk factor because there are more heart problems among older people.**
  1. As people get older risk factors tend to be manifest or induced:
     a. less physical activity
     b. poor nutrition
     c. obesity
  2. However, the process begins early in life:
     a. young people should not think they are escaping
     b. autopsies conducted on young soldiers in Korea and Vietnam revealed that approximately 70% had early stages of atherosclerosis
     c. other studies have found elevated blood cholesterol levels in children as young as 10 years old

B. **Even though aging cannot be stopped, it can be slowed down:**
  1. Physiological versus chronological age is an important concept in preventing disease.
  2. Some individuals in their 60s or older have the body of a 20-year-old.
  3. Some 20-year-olds seem to have the body of a 60-year-old.

C. **Risk factor management and positive lifestyles habits are the best ways to slow down the natural aging process.**

XIII. FINAL WORD FOR CORONARY RISK REDUCTION

A. **Most of the risk factors for CHD are reversible and preventable.**

B. **Person and family history risk factors does not mean this person is doomed.**

C. **A healthier lifestyle is something over which you have much control.**

D. **Will power, commitment, and persistence are required to develop patterns that eventually will turn into healthy habits contributing to total well-being.**

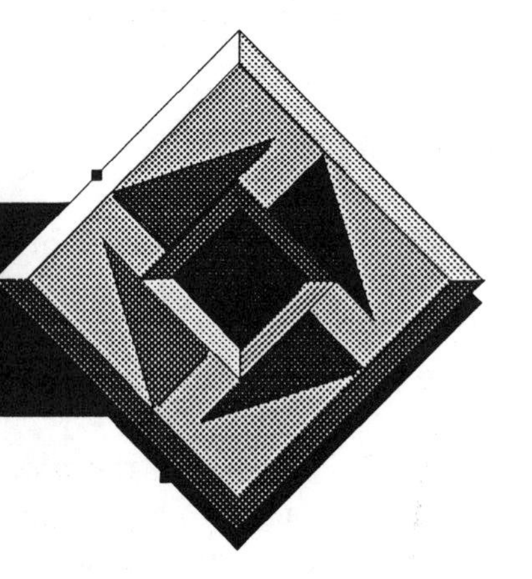

Instructor Activities

1. **Show overhead transparency 52** (from the color transparency packet) to contrast a normal healthy heart and a myocardial infarction. Show how the coronary arteries provide the tissues of the heart muscle with oxygen and nutrients.

2. **Show overhead transparency 9-1** in this manual and discuss disorders of the vessels related to heart attack, stroke, and hypertension. Distinguish between a normal artery, an artery occluded by atherosclerotic plaque, and an artery hardened by arterosclerosis. Differentiate between an embolism and a thrombus. Explain how these vascular disorders gradually develop over years. Also explain how aneurysms, tumors, and vascular spasms can interfere with bloodflow to the heart and brain.

3. **Show overhead transparency 9-2** and contrast situations A, B, and C. Situation A is a healthy heart with clean, smooth coronary artery walls and with well developed collateral circulation. B is an occluded coronary artery on a person whose heart was pretty healthy. Because the arteries were fairly large, only a small part of the heart was deprived of oxygen and the person survived. C shows a massive occlusion blocking the flow of oxygen to a large part of the heart. Survival is unlikely.

4. **Show overhead transparency 9-3** and discuss interrelationship among the leading cardiovascular risk factors. Distinguish between the risk factors that can't be changed and the risk factors that can be changed. Then explain what can be done in each of the areas of involving lifestyle behaviors to promote cardiovascular wellness.

5. **Show overhead transparency 9-4** to explain the role of cholesterol in the body, to distinguish between HDLs and LDLs, and to help students understand what they can do to maintain a healthy cholesterol profile.

6. **Show overhead transparency 9-5** to explain how blood pressure is taken, the meaning of the values, the detrimental effect of high blood pressure, and what a person should do to control blood pressure.

7. **Show overhead transparency 9-6** surgical procedures for coronary occlusion.

8. **Show overhead transparency 9-7** showing the incidence of cardiovascular disease in the United States for selected years from 1900 to 1990. Emphasize the improvement that has taken place since 1960. Point out that most of the risk factors are preventable and reversible.

VASCULAR DISORDERS

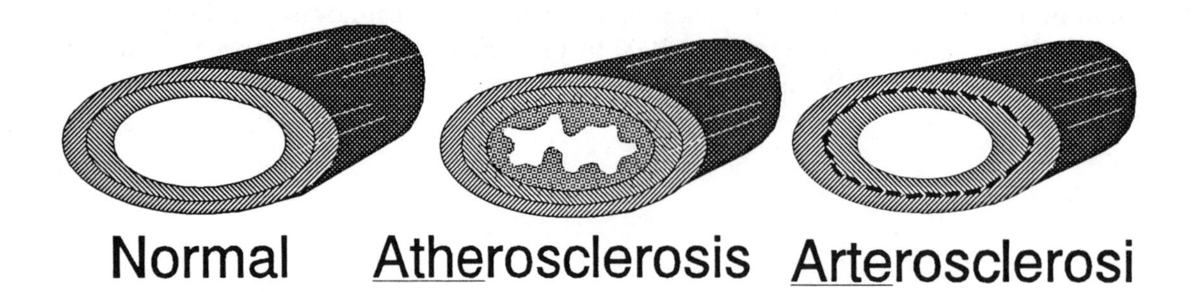

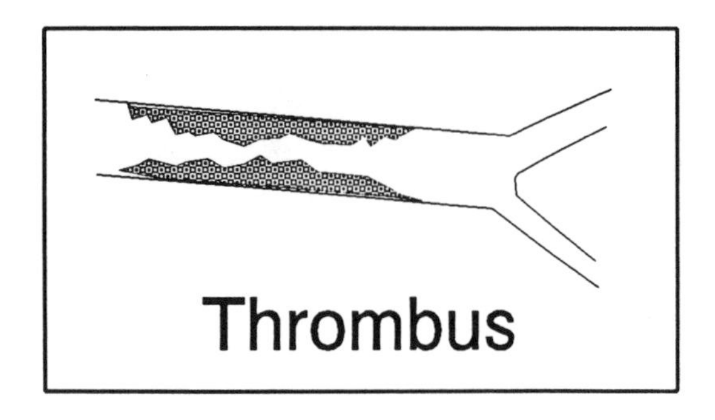

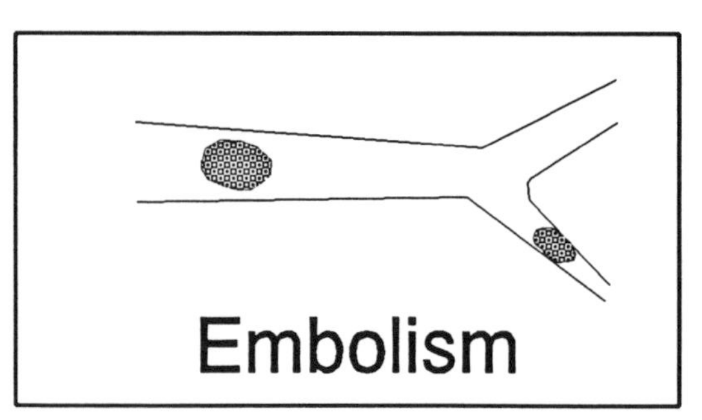

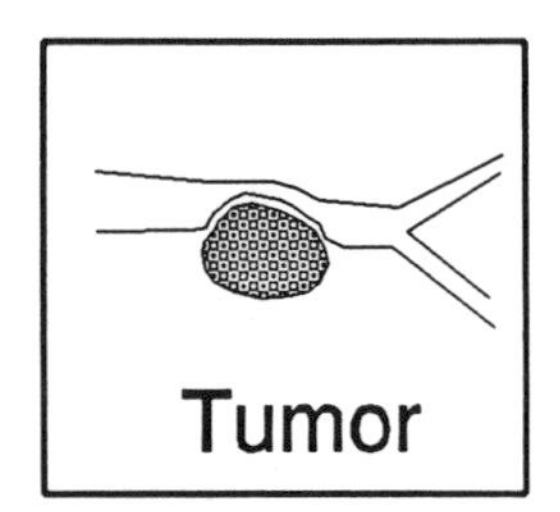

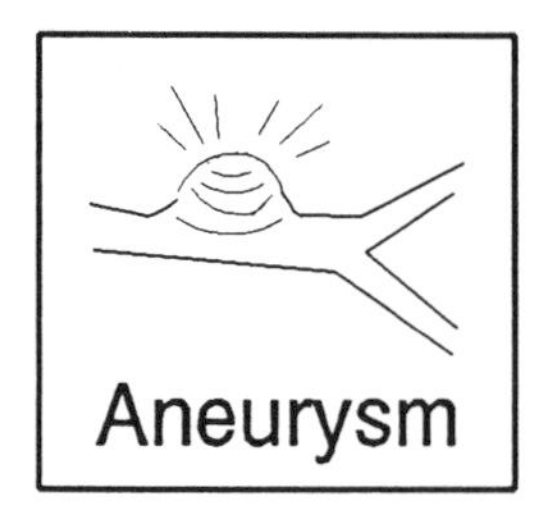

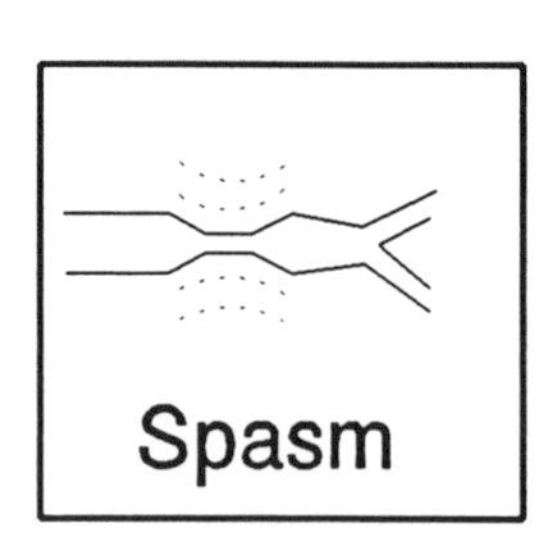

HEART ATTACK | STROKE | HYPERTENSION

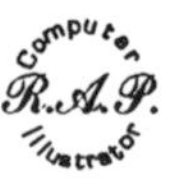

9-1

HEALTHY HEART

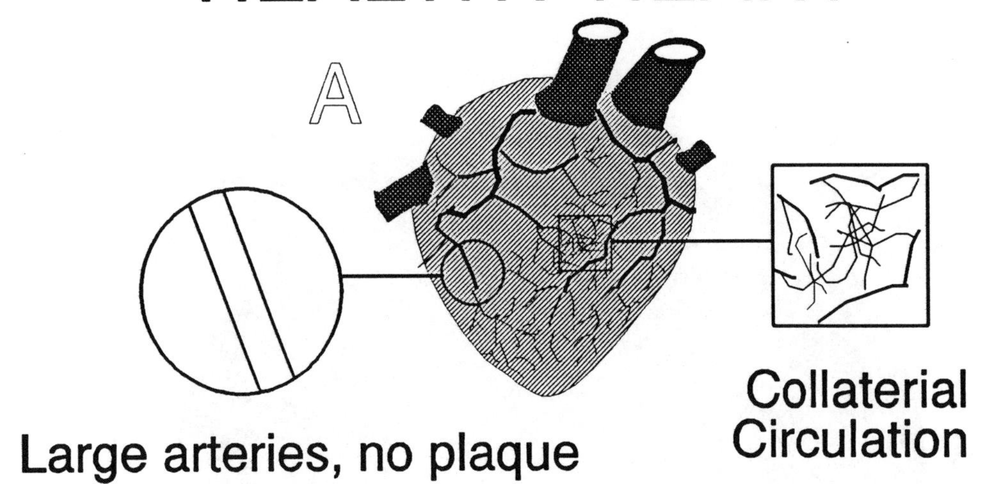

HEART ATTACK

Coronary Occlusion

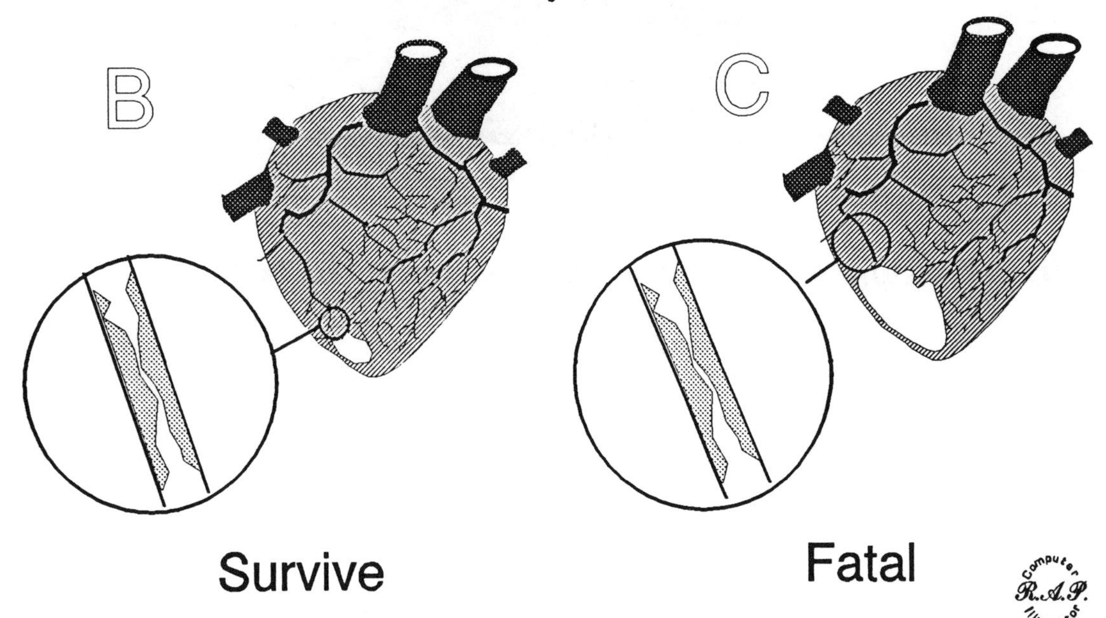

9-2

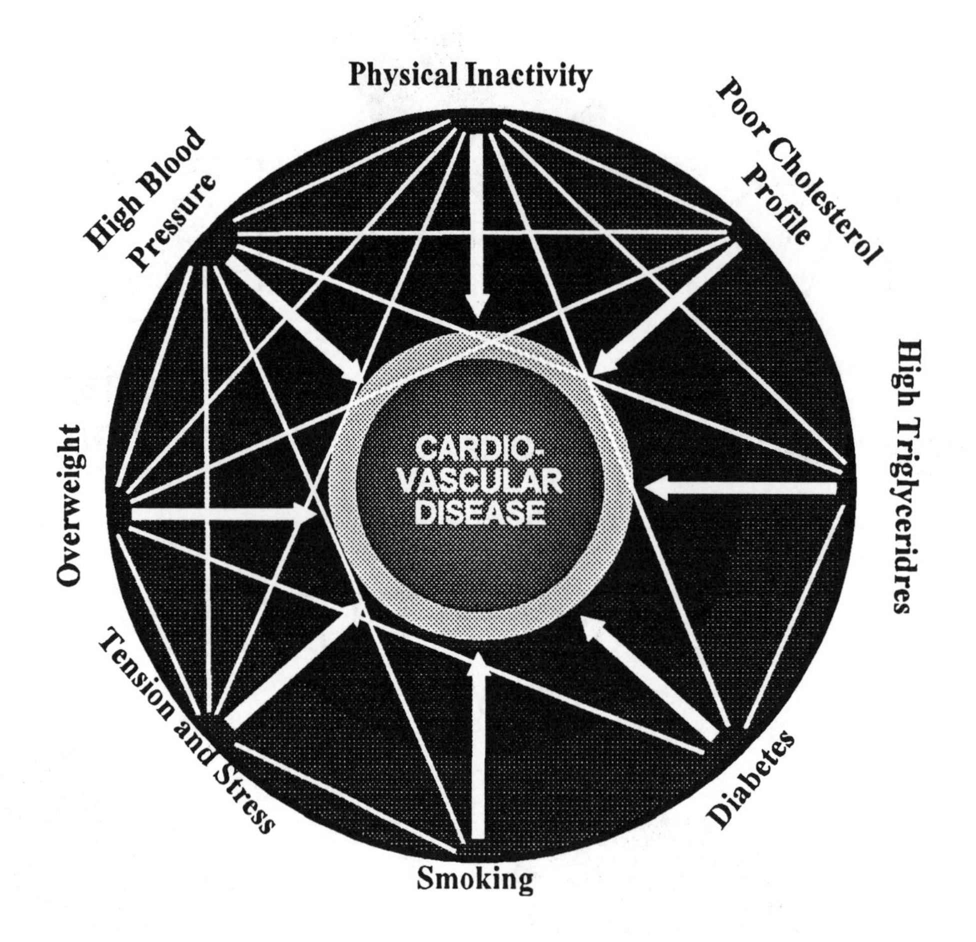

Interrelationships among leading cardiovascular risk factors.

9-3

Cholesterol Guidelines	Amount	Rating
Total Cholesterol	<200 mg/dl 200-239 mg/dl >240 mg/dl	Desirable Borderline High risk
LDL-Cholesterol	<130 mg/dl 130-159 mg/dl >160 mg/dl	Desirable Borderline High risk
HDL-Cholesterol	>45 mg/dl 36-44 mg/dl >35 mg/dl	Desirable Borderline High risk

Triglycerides Guidelines	Amount	Rating
	>125 mg/dl 126-499 mg/dl >500 mg/dl	Desirable Borderline High risk

Blood Glucose Guidelines	Amount	Rating
	>120 121-159 >160	Desirable Borderline High risk

Blood Pressure Guidelines		
Rating	**Systolic**	**Diastolic**
Ideal Borderline high Hypertension	<120 121-139 >140	<80 mmHg 81-89 mmHg >90 mmHg

9-4

BLOOD PRESSURE

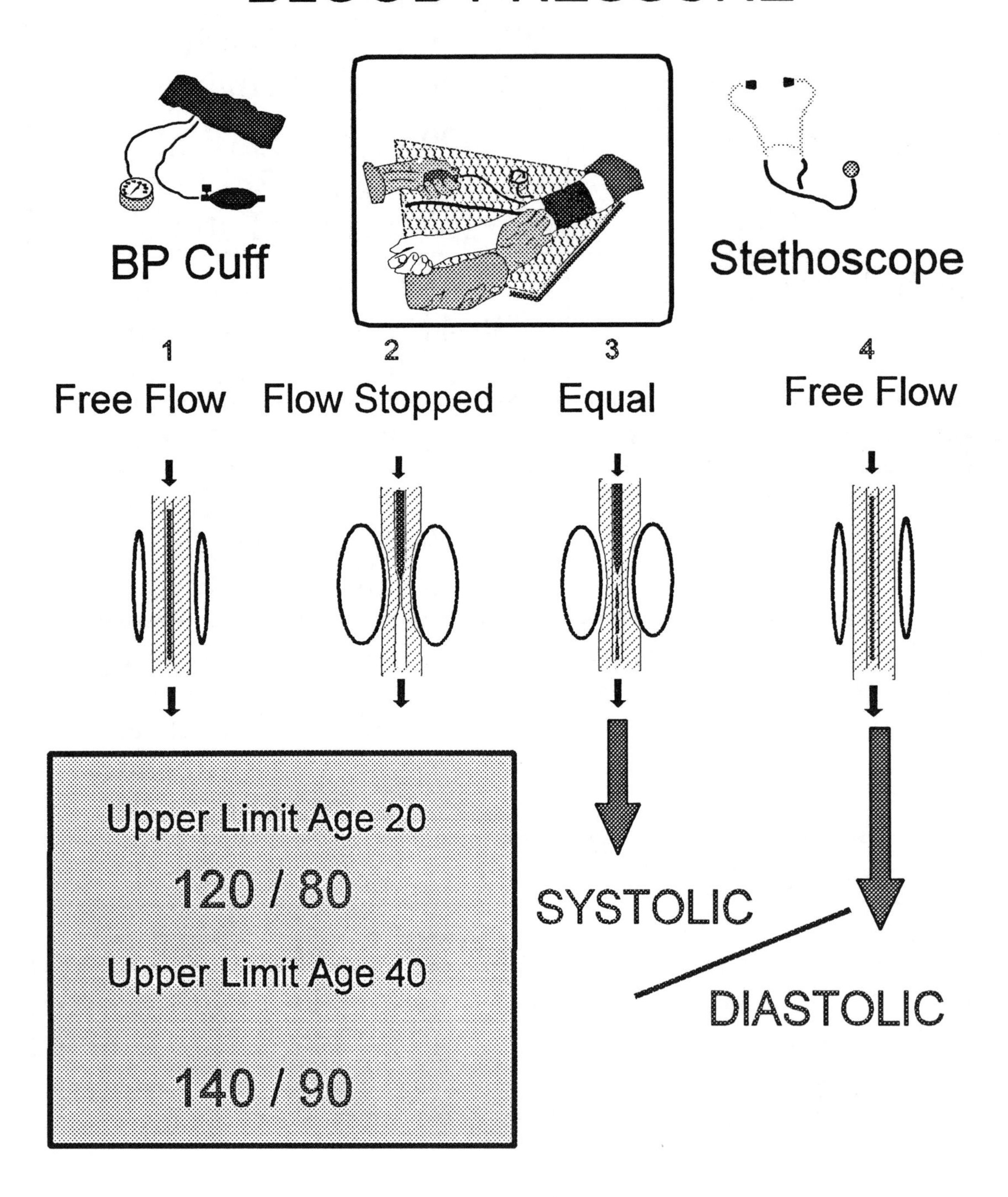

9-5

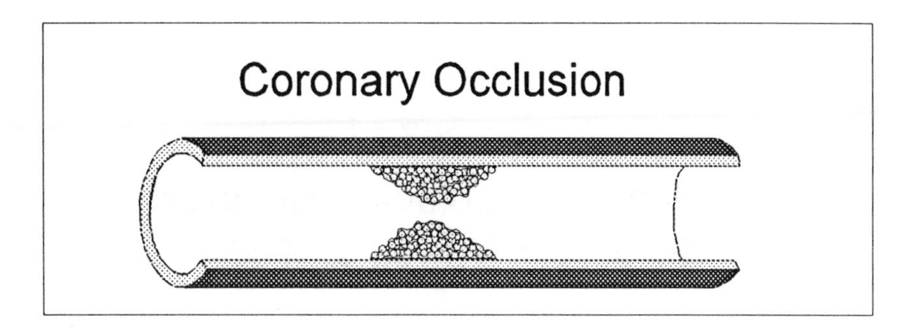

Surgical Procedures for Coronary Occlusion

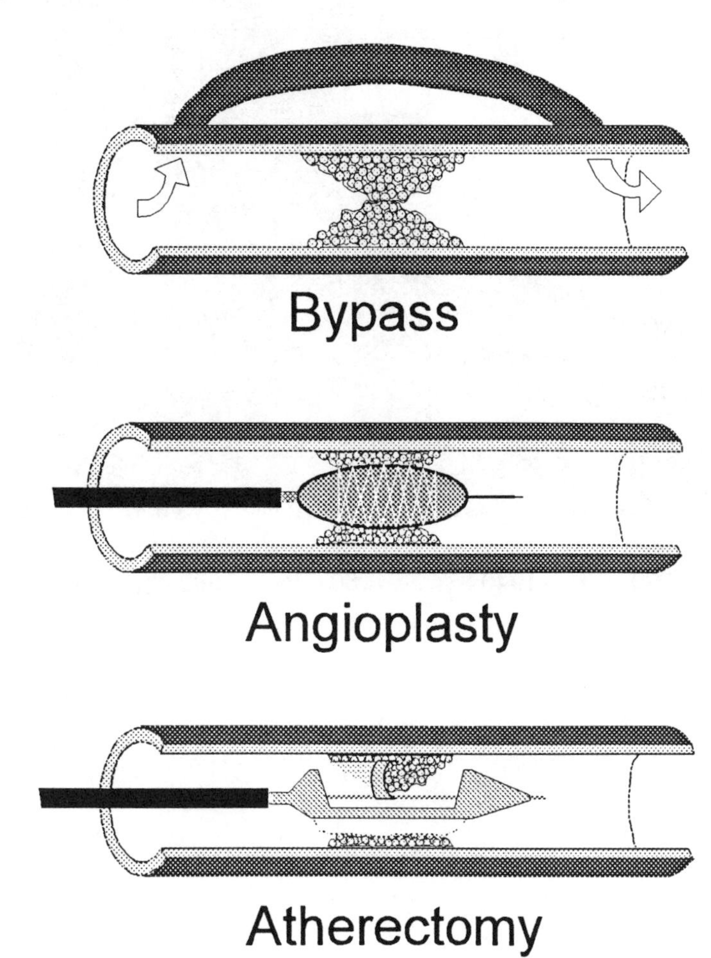

12-3

9-6

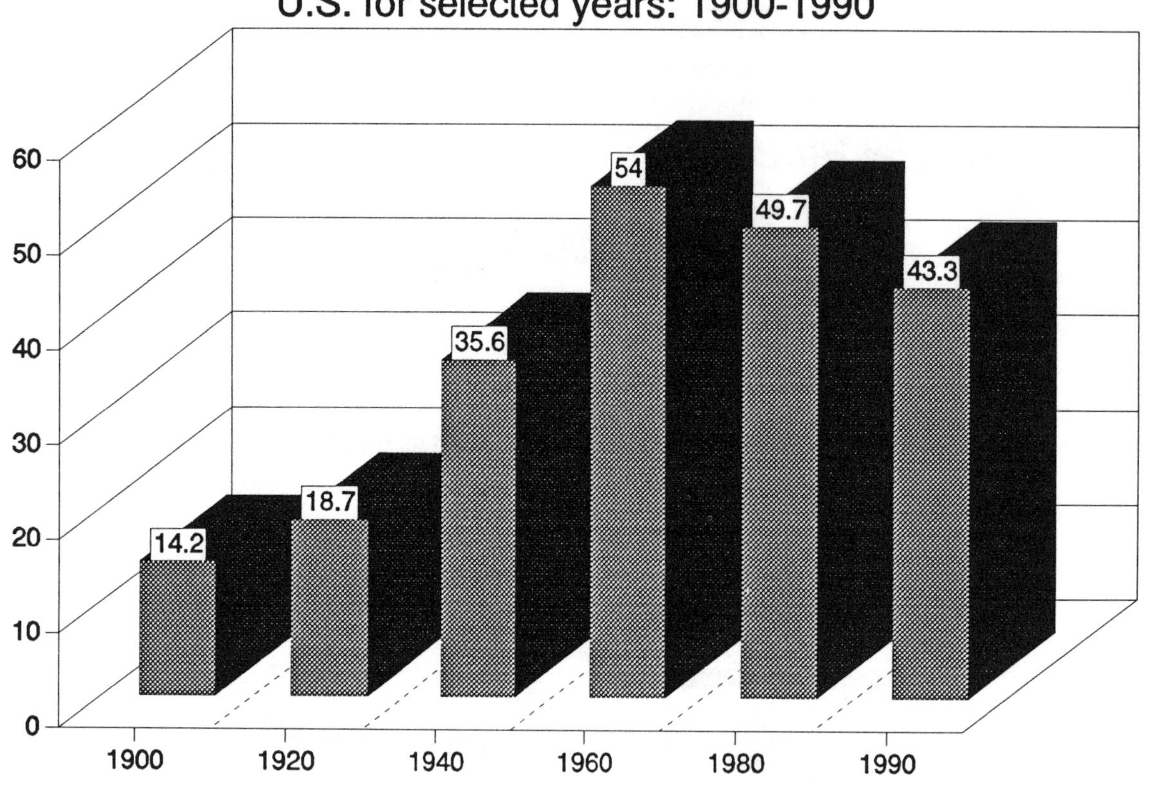
Incidence of cardiovascular disease
U.S. for selected years: 1900-1990
60
50
40
30
20
10
0
14.2
18.7
35.6
54
49.7
43.3
1900
1920
1940
1960
1980
1990

9-7

Cancer Risk Management

1

Expanded Chapter Outline

I. INTRODUCTION

A. The 100 trillion cells in the human body normally reproduce themselves in an orderly way:

1. The cell growth has to take place so old, worn-out tissue can be replaced and injuries can be repaired.
2. Cell growth is controlled by DNA and RNA genetic codes found in the nucleus of each cell.

B. Cells that grow abnormally and form a mass of tissue are called a tumor:

1. Benign tumors do not invade other tissues.
2. A malignant tumor is a cancer which invades other tissues and causes death.

C. A cancer begins with an alteration in DNA codes in a cell:

1. Cancer genes and suppressor genes are found within the DNA.
2. They normally work together to repair and replace cells.
   a. cancer genes (oncogenes) initiate cell division.
   b. suppressor genes deactivate the process.
3. Normally in cell division, the DNA molecule is duplicated perfectly.
4. Sometimes the DNA molecule is not replicated exactly:
   a. usually cells with defective DNA will die.
   b. occasionally they continue dividing and form a tumor.
5. Defects in these cells allow the cell to grow into a malignant tumor or cancer.
6. These defects or mutations may be caused by:
   a. external factors -- radiation, chemicals, and viruses.
   b. internal factors -- immune conditions, hormones, and mutations.

7. A decade or more can pass between the mutations and the time cancer is diagnosed.

D. Recent discoveries (1994) have found that abnormal cell division is related to strands of molecules (telomeres) found at both ends of a chromosome.

1. Each time a cell divides, chromosomes lose some telomeres.
2. After many cell divisions, chromosomes eventually run out of telomeres and the cell dies (this may be associates with the aging process).
3. Human tumors, however, make an enzyme known as telomerase.
4. Telomerase keep the chromosomes from running out of telomeres.
5. This allows cancer cells to reproduce indefinitely.

E. Cancer starts with the abnormal growth of one cell, which multiplies rapidly.

1. At about a million cells it is referred to as carcinoma in situ.
2. This is a critical point, it is encapsulated and has not started to spread.
3. To grow, the tumor requires more oxygen and nutrients.
4. In time cancer cells produce chemicals that enhance capillary formation into the tumor (angiogenesis).
5. Angiogenesis is the precursor of metastasis.
6. Through these new vessels, cancer cells can break away from a malignant tumor, migrate to other parts of the body, and there start new cancers.

F. While encapsulated, the tumor may go without significant growth.

1. It may remain undetected for months or years.
2. At this point it does not pose a serious threat to human health.
3. By middle age most adults have cancerous cells in their bodies.
4. The immune system destroys most cancerous cells.
5. However, if only one abnormal cell survives it may be deadly.
6. The rate at which cancer cells grow varies from one type to another.
7. Once cancer cells metastasize, treatment becomes more difficult.

G. Therapy can kill most cancer cells.

1. However, some cells may become resistant to treatment.
2. These cells can produce tumors that are resistant to the treatment.

II. INCIDENCE OF CANCER

A. Cancer is the second leading killer in this country.

1. In 1990 cancer was the cause of 23.5% of all deaths in the U.S.
2. More than half a million Americans die from cancer each year.
3. 1 in 3 Americans alive today eventually will be diagnosed with cancer.
4. Those figures could be reduced dramatically through lifestyle changes.

B. Cancer is largely preventable.

1. 80% of all cancer is related to lifestyle or environmental factors.
2. These factors include:
   a. diet
   b. tobacco use
   c. excessive use of alcohol
   d. sexual and reproductive history
   e. exposure to occupational hazards
3. Individuals who have a healthy lifestyle have lower cancer death rates.

C. Because of better detection and treatment methods, more than 8 million Americans with a history of cancer were alive in 1993:
1. Nearly 5 million of whom were considered cured.
2. For most patients, "cured" means 5 years without symptoms after treatments stop.
3. Life expectancy for these individuals is the same as for those who never have had cancer.

III. GUIDELINES FOR CANCER PREVENTION

A. The biggest factor in fighting cancer today is health education.
1. People need to be informed about the:
   a. risk factors for cancer
   b. guidelines for early detection.
2. The most effective way to protect against cancer is to change negative lifestyle habits and behaviors.

B. DIET
1. The diet should:
   a. be low in fat
   b. be high in fiber
   c. contain vitamins A and C from natural sources
   d. keep protein intake within the RDA guidelines
   e. include cruciferous vegetables (plants with cross-shaped leaves)
   f. avoid alcohol or use it in moderation
   g. avoid obesity

2. Fat and fiber:
   a. high fat intake has been linked primarily to breast, colon, and prostate cancers.
   b. low intake of fiber seems to increase the risk for colon cancer.
3. Vitamins A and C:
   a. foods high in vitamin A and C may deter larynx, esophagus, and lung cancers.
   b. vitamin C seems to discourage the formation of cancer-causing substances formed from eating cured meats.
   c. beta-carotene (a precursor to vitamin A) and vitamin C. found in cruciferous

vegetables seem to protect against cancer.
   (1) carrots, squash, sweet potatoes, cauliflower, broccoli, cabbage, brussels sprouts, and kohlrabi.
   (2) researchers believe the antioxidant effect of these vitamins protects the body from oxygen free radicals.

4. Phytochemicals:
   a. a promising concept in cancer prevention.
   b. are found in fruits and vegetables.
   c. appear to block and disrupt the formation and development of cancerous tumors:
      (1) removing carcinogens from cells before they cause damage.
      (2) activating enzymes that detoxify cancer-causing agents.
      (3) keeping carcinogens from locking onto cells.
      (4) preventing carcinogens from binding to DNA.
      (5) breaking up cancer-causing precursors to benign forms.
      (6) disrupting the chemical combination of cell molecules that can produce carcinogens.
      (7) Kkeping small tumors from accessing capillaries to get oxygen and nutrients.
   d. As examples of phytochemicals:
      (1) sulforaphane in broccoli
      (2) PEITC in broccoli
      (3) capsaicin in hot chili peppers
      (4) genistein in soybeans
      (5) flavenoids in most fruits and vegetables
      (6) P-coumaric and chlorogenic acids in strawberries, green peppers, tomatoes, and pineapples
5. Nutritional guidelines also recommend avoiding excessive protein:
   a. daily protein intake for some Americans is almost twice the amount the human body needs.
   b. too much animal protein seems to decrease blood enzymes that prevent precancerous cells from developing into tumors.
   c. grilling protein at high temperatures for a long time may increase the formation of carcinogenic substances.
   d. some suggestions for barbecuing meat include:
      (1) microwaving the meat for a couple of minutes first, but do not use the fluids.
      (2) removing the skin before serving.
      (3) cooking at lower heat to medium rather than well done.
6. Alcohol should be consumed in moderation, if at all.
   a. too much alcohol raises the risk for developing certain cancers, especially when it is combined with tobacco.
   b. in combination, these substances significantly increase the risk for mouth, larynx, throat, esophagus, and liver cancers.
   c. the combined action of heavy use of alcohol and tobacco increases cancer of

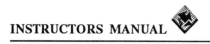

the oral cavity.

7. Body Weight:
   a. maintaining recommended body weight also is encouraged.
   b. obesity has been associated with cancers of the colon, rectum, breast, prostate, gallbladder, ovary, and uterus.

C. Abstaining From Tobacco

1. Smoking is also linked to 30% of all cancers.
   a. smoking is the culprit in 83% of lung cancers.
   b. smokeless tobacco also increases the risk for mouth, larynx, throat, and esophagus cancers.
   c. about 138,600 cancer deaths each year stem from tobacco use.
2. Cigarette smoking by itself is a major health hazard:
   a. when considering all related deaths, cigarette smoking is responsible for about 418,000 unnecessary deaths each year.
   b. the average life expectancy for a chronic smoker is up to 18 years less than for a nonsmoker.

D. Avoiding Excessive Sun Exposure

1. Too much exposure to sunlight (including tanning booths) is a major contributor to skin cancer:
   a. The most common sites of skin cancer are those exposed to the sun most often (face, neck, and back of the hands).
   b. The three types of skin cancer are:
      (1) basal cell carcinoma
      (2) squamous cell carcinoma
      (3) malignant melanoma
   c. Melanoma is the most deadly, causing approximately 6,900 deaths in 1993.
   d. Most skin cancer cases could have been prevented by protecting the skin from the sun's rays.
   e. One in six Americans will develop some type of skin cancer.
2. Nothing is healthy about a "healthy tan."
   a. Even small doses of sunlight add up to a greater risk for skin cancer and premature aging.
   b. The tan fades at the end of the summer season, but the underlying skin damage does not disappear.
   c. Vitamin B rays (UVB) are thought to be the main cause of premature wrinkling, skin aging, and skin cancer.
   d. Unfortunately, the damage may not become evident until up to 20 years later.
3. People with sensitive skin should avoid sun exposure between 10:00 a.m. and 3:00 p.m.
4. Sunscreen lotions should be used:
   a. They should be applied about 30 minutes before exposure.
   b. The skin takes that long to absorb the protective ingredients.
   c. A sun protection factor (SPF) of at least 15 is recommended.

(1) SPF 15 means the skin takes 15 times longer to burn than with no lotion.
(2) if you ordinarily get a mild sunburn after 20 minutes of noonday sun, an SPF 15 allows you to remain in the sun about 300 minutes before burning.
(3) the higher the number, the more the protection.

d. When swimming or sweating sunscreens should be reapplied more often.

E. Estrogen, Radiation Exposure, and Potential Occupational Hazards

1. Estrogen intake has been linked to endometrial cancer but can be taken safely under careful supervision by a physician.
2. Although radiation exposure increases the risk for cancer, the benefits of x-rays may outweigh the risk involved when precautions are taken to minimize the possible dose.
3. Exposure to certain occupational hazards increase the risk of cancer:
    a. such substances include asbestos fibers, nickel and uranium dusts, chromium compounds, vinyl chloride, and ether,
    b. appropriate safety precautions should be followed.
    c. cigarette smoking magnifies the risk from occupational hazards.

F. Physical Activity

1. A more active lifestyle and lower stress levels also seem to offer a protective effect against cancer.
2. A moderately intense lifetime exercise program has been shown to lower the risk for cancers of the breast, colon, and reproductive system.
3. The body's autoimmune system may play a role in preventing cancer and exercise improves the autoimmune system.

IV. EARLY DETECTION

A. Fortunately, through early detection many cancers can be controlled or cured.

B. Everyone should become familiar with the following seven warning signals for cancer and bring them to a physician's attention if any are present:

1. Change in bowel or bladder habits.
2. Sore that does not heal.
3. Unusual bleeding or discharge.
4. Thickening or lump in breast or elsewhere.
5. Indigestion or difficulty in swallowing.
6. Obvious change in wart or mole.
7. Nagging cough or hoarseness.

C. The questionnaire at the end of this chapter should alert people to cancer symptoms. Any of the symptoms calls for a physician's attention as soon as possible.

D. The Guidelines for Screening Recommendations by the American Cancer Society

(Table 10.1) should be included in regular physical examinations.

E. **Treatment of cancer always should be left to specialized physicians and cancer clinics.**

F. **Current treatment modalities include:**
1. surgery
2. radiation
3. radioactive substances
4. chemotherapy
5. hormones
6. immunotherapy

V. TYPES OF CANCER

A. CARCINOMAS:
1. Affect the tissues that line most body cavities and that cover body surfaces.
   a. The most common kind of cancers
   b. Spread through the bloodstream and lymph system
2. Examples are cancers of the lung, breast, skin, colon, uterus.

B. SARCOMAS:
1. Affect the connective tissues of the body
   a. less common than carcinomas, but they grow and spread more quickly
   b. spread through the bloodstream
2. Examples are sarcomas of the muscles, bones, and cartilage.

C. LYMPHOMAS:
1. Lymphomas are cancers of the lymphatic, or infection-fighting, cells.
   a. lymph nodes in the groin, armpits, and neck can be affected
   b. spread through the lymph system
2. An example of lymphoma is Hodgkin's disease.

D. MELANOMAS:
1. Affect the skin.
   a. grow and spread rapidly
   b. spread through the bloodstream
2. They generally begin as a mole that later becomes cancerous.

E. LEUKEMIA:
1. Leukemia affect the tissues that manufacture blood.
   a. especially the spleen and the bone marrow
   b. spread through the bloodstream

F. NEUROBLASTOMAS:

1. Affect the nervous system or the adrenal glands.
    a. relatively uncommon
    b. spread through the bloodstream
2. They occur most often in children under age 10.

VI. SITES OF CANCER

A. LUNG CANCER:

1. is the leading cancer killer.
    a. it afflicts approximately 157,000 Americans each year.
    b. approximately 142,000 of them die.
2. Lung cancer occurs almost exclusively among cigarette smokers:
    a. sexual differences:
        (1) once cancer was a disease predominantly affecting men.
        (2) now the leading cause of death from cancer among women.
        (3) has risen along with increased smoking rates among women.
        (4) is steadily decreasing in men and steadily increasing in women.
3. Lung cancer spreads rapidly, and it is rarely detected early:
    a. usually does not cause early symptoms
    b. does not show up on an x-ray until it is quite advanced.
    c. by that time, damage is usually too extensive to treat successfully.
4. Risks:
    a. cigarette smoking is the number-one risk factor
    b. secondary smoke also significantly increases the risk
    c. other risk factors are much higher if the individual also smokes.
    d. other risk factors for lung cancer include exposure to:
        (1) asbestos
        (2) severe air pollution
        (3) carcinogenic chemicals
        (4) certain metals
        (5) arsenic or radioactive ores.
        (6) radon gas.

B. COLON AND RECTAL CANCER:

1. Colon and rectum cancer is the second leading cancer killer:
    a. about 155,000 new cases are diagnosed each year
    b. almost 60,000 Americans die of colorectal cancer annually
2. If detected early, colorectal cancer usually can be treated successfully.
3. It grows and spreads quite slowly.
4. Signs and symptoms include:
    a. bleeding from the rectum--bright red blood in the stools
    b. a change in bowel habits can indicate colorectal cancer
5. Risk factors include:
    a. personal or family history of polyps in the colon or rectum.

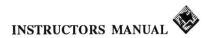

b. family history of colorectal cancer
c. diet high in fats and low in fiber
d. inflammatory bowel problems (such as colitis)
e. age (after 40) is also considered a risk factor
f. high-fat, low-fiber diet

C. SKIN CANCER:
1. Accounts for approximately 40% of all cancers.
   a. more than half a million new diagnosed cases every year
   b. approximately 8,000 deaths annually
2. The three basic kinds of skin cancers are:
   a. **Basal cell carcinoma.**
      (1) the most common and least serious form of the skin cancers
      (2) it usually does not spread, and it grows slowly
      (3) most occur on areas of sun exposure--face, neck, hands
      (4) easily detected and treated
   b. **Squamous cell carcinoma:**
      (1) grows faster than the basal cell type
      (2) involves deeper layers of skin
      (3) rarely spreads to other parts of the body
      (4) easily detected and treated
   c. **Malignant melanoma:**
      (1) the most dangerous skin cancer--6,000 deaths each year
      (2) a rapidly growing cancer
      (3) almost always spreads to other organs.
      (4) can be treated successfully if it is diagnosed and treated early
3. The risk factors for skin cancer include:
   a. sun exposure (the strongest is between 10 a.m. and 2 p.m.)
   b. fair skin that burns easily and rarely tans
   c. fair skin that sometimes tans
   d. blonde or red hair
   e. artificial sources of ultraviolet rays, such as tanning booths
   f. history of one or more severe sunburns
   g. a dark brown or black wart
   h. birthmarks or congenital moles
   i. moles that are irritated chronically
   j. occupational exposure to creosote, coal tar, pitch, arsenic, or radium
4. The sharp increase in skin cancers has researchers alarmed:
   a. they are concerned about the gradual deterioration of the ozone layer
   b. researchers believe tanning habits are at fault, young women have twice the rate as young men

D. BREAST CANCER:
1. The second leading killer of women.
   a. kills almost 50,000 American women each year

   b. one in nine women will develop breast cancer
2. Early detection is the key to successful treatment and improved survival rates.
   a. heightened awareness of the disease
   b. breast self-examination
   c. regular mammogram
3. General symptoms of breast cancer include:
   a. a thickening or lump in the breast
   b. distortion or dimpling of a breast
   c. swollen lymph nodes under the arm
   d. retraction, pain, discharge, or scaliness of the nipple
4. General risk factors for breast cancer include:
   a. a grandmother, mother, or sister with breast cancer
   b. early onset of menstruation (before age 12)
   c. delayed onset of menopause (after age 55)
   d. first pregnancy after age 30
   e. obesity
   f. a woman who has never been pregnant
   g. a woman who has never breast-fed
   h. age (dramatic increase after age 50)
5. Questionable risk factors:
   a. hormone replacement therapy and oral contraceptives?
   b. diet?
   c. breast Feeding?
   d. known risk factors account for a small percentage of breast cancer, the majority of patients (60%-70%) have no known risk factors.

E. CERVICAL CANCER:
1. Approximately 60,000 women are diagnosed with invasive cervical cancer each year in the United States.
2. The death rate from cancer of the cervix has decreased significantly:
   a. the rate went down more than 70% during the past four decades.
   b. this is because of early detection through:
      (1) Pap smears
      (2) regular gynecological examinations.
3. With early diagnosis, treatment usually is successful.
   a. recognizing early symptoms is important.
   b. unusual vaginal bleeding or discharge is often an early symptom.
4. Risk factors for cervical cancer can be:
   a. early age at first intercourse.
   b. multiple sex partners.
   c. a history of viral genital infections.
   d. cigarette smoking.
   e. the human papilloma virus can cause cervical cancer.
      (1) it is a sexually transmitted virus
      (2) it is responsible for genital warts

F. UTERINE CANCER:

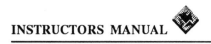

1. Cancer of the uterus affects about 48,000 women in the U.S. each year.
2. Only about 4,000 deaths a year are attributed to uterine cancer.
3. The death rate from uterine cancer has fallen dramatically.
4. With early detection, treatment generally is successful.
5. Symptoms of uterine cancer might be:
   a. unusual vaginal discharge
   b. unusual vaginal bleeding
   c. bleeding between menstrual periods
6. Risk factors for uterine cancer include:
   a. late onset of menopause
   b. history of infertility
   c. prolonged estrogen replacement therapy
   d. obesity
   e. diabetes

G. OVARIAN CANCER:

1. Ovarian cancer claims about 13,000 American women each year.
2. It is a particularly difficult cancer to diagnose and treat.
   a. it reveals no symptoms until in its latest stages
   b. the five year survival rate averages 40%
3. Late symptoms include:
   a. abdominal swelling or bloating
   b. persistent abdominal gas
   c. unexplained stomachaches or indigestion
4. Factors include:
   a. age, it is highest for women in their 60s
   b. race, rates are higher among Jewish women, Americans, Scandinavians, and Scots
   c. a grandmother, mother, or sister with ovarian cancer
   d. never had children (doubles the risk)
   e. use of oral contraceptives
   f. occurrence of colorectal, breast, or uterine cancer (doubles the risk)
   g. early onset of ovulation

H. PROSTATE CANCER:

1. Prostrate cancer is the leading cancer in American men:
   a. the third leading cause of cancer death in men
   b. strikes more than 160,000 men in the U.S. every year
   c. more than 30,000 die from it
2. Prostate cancer often is detected early:
   a. provokes an array of early symptoms
   b. symptoms are often mistaken for other ailments
3. If detected early, it can be treated successfully about 84% of the time.

4. A new blood test, prostate-specific antigen (PSA), can be used to help diagnose prostate cancer.
5. Signs and symptoms of prostate cancer include:
   a. pain in the pelvis, lower back, or upper thighs
   b. blood in the urine or semen
   c. pain or burning during urination
   d. unusual urination patterns
      (1) frequent urination
      (2) weak or interrupted urine flow
      (3) difficulty starting or stopping urine flow
      (4) inability to urinate
6. Risk factors for prostate cancer include:
   a. age, most are after age 65
   b. race, African-American men have the highest rate in the world
   c. a family history of prostate cancer
   d. occupational exposure to cadmium
   e. a high-fat diet

I. TESTICULAR CANCER:

1. This is the most common cancer in men between ages 15 and 34.
2. The incidence in this age group has been increasing steadily.
3. The chances for cure are nearly 100% if found early.
4. Many men discover the cancer themselves through self-examination.
5. The warning signs are:
   a. a painless thickening or hard lump in the testicle
   b. an accumulation of fluid or blood in the scrotum
   c. a dull ache in the groin that may involve the lower abdomen
6. Risk factors for testicular cancer include:
   a. an undescended testicle after age 6
   b. a grandfather, father, or brother with testicular cancer

J. PANCREATIC CANCER:

1. There are more than 70,000 new cases each year.
2. More than 25,000 Americans die from pancreatic cancer each year.
3. The incidence of pancreatic cancer has doubled in the past two decades.
4. It is the fifth most common cancer killer in Americans.
5. The survival rate from pancreatic cancer is low.
   a. the disease spreads rapidly
   b. few survive more than 3 years
6. Pancreatic cancer is a *silent* disease, progressing without symptoms.
7. Risk factors include:
   a. age, the highest risk is between ages 65 and 79
   b. sex, men are at higher risk
   c. race, African-Americans are at higher risk
   d. smoking cigarettes

e. consuming alcohol
f. eating a high-fat diet
g. being exposed to gasoline and some chemical cleaners on the job

K. **KIDNEY AND BLADDER CANCER:**
1. There are approximately 50,000 new cases in the U.S. each year.
2. Close to 10,000 Americans die from it each year.
3. Almost nine in 10 can be cured if detected early.
4. The most common signs of bladder cancer are:
   a. more frequent urination
   b. blood in the urine
5. Risk factors include:
   a. sex, it is four times more common in men than in women
   b. cigarette smoking
   c. occupational exposure to leather and rubber
   d. occupational exposure to dyes
   e. living in an urban area

L. **ORAL CANCER:**
1. More than 30,000 Americans are diagnosed with oral cancer each year.
2. Approximately 8,500 die from it.
3. Oral cancer has increased substantially over the past two decades.
   a. the increase correlates with the popularity of smokeless tobacco
   b. twice as many men as women get oral cancer
4. Signs of oral cancer generally include:
   a. a sore that fails to heal or that bleeds easily
   b. a reddish or whitish patch that does not go away
   c. a lump or thickening in the cheek, tongue, or lips
   d. difficulty chewing or swallowing
5. Risk factors include:
   a. use of smokeless tobacco (chewing tobacco)
   b. smoking cigarettes, cigars, or a pipe
   c. excessive alcohol consumption

M. **OTHER CANCER SITES:**
1. Lymphomas--cancer of the lymphatic system.
2. Leukemia--cancer that interferes with blood-forming tissues (bone marrow, lymph nodes, and spleen), by producing too many immature white blood cells.
3. Liver Cancer--The incidence in the United States is very low. Men are more prone than women, and the disease is more common after age sixty.
4. Thyroid Cancer--The thyroid gland is located in the lower portion of the front of the neck, helps regulate growth and metabolism. Thyroid cancer occurs almost twice as often in women as in men.
5. Esophageal and Stomach Cancer--The incidence of gastric cancer in the United States has dropped about 40 percent in the last thirty years. This type of cancer is

more common in men.

VII. WHAT CAN YOU DO?

A. An ounce of prevention is worth a pound of cure.

B. Although cardiovascular disease is the number-one killer in the country, more people fear cancer.

C. Of all cancers, 60% to 80% are preventable, and about 50% are curable.

D. Most cancers are lifestyle-related.

E. Being aware of the risk factors and general recomendations and following the screening guidelines will greatly help.

WHAT ARE YOUR CHANCES ?

Based on the U.S. average for all types of cancer:

Of every 100 people, 33 will get cancer.

Of those 33, approximately 15 will survive
and 18 will die.

Of the 18 who died, at least **4** more could have survived
if the cancer had been detected and treated in time.

Much of the effort in cancer education

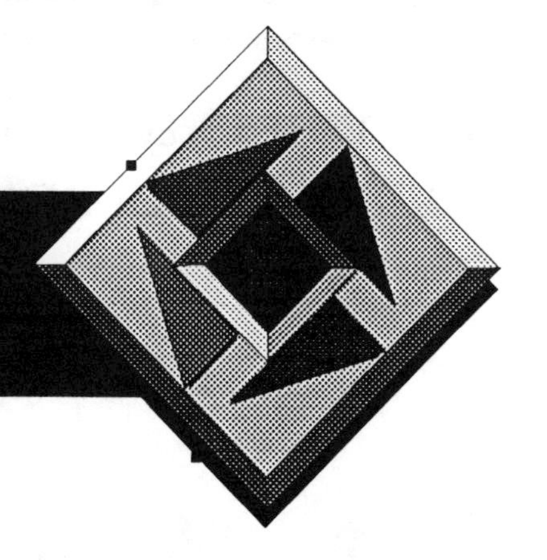

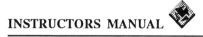

Instructor Activities

1. **Show overhead transparency** 10-1 to answer the question, What is Cancer. Outline the characteristics of the family of diseases called cancer. Diferentiate among the following types of cancer: Carcinomas, Sarcomas, Lymphomas, Melanomas, Leukemias, and Neuroblastomas.

2. **Show overhead transparency** 10-2 to to further answer the question, What is cancer. Diferentiate between benign and maliginant tumors. Explain that cancers spread into local tissues and to other parts of the body through a proscess called metastasis.

3. **Show overhead transparency** 61 (from the color transparency packet) to show another illustration of how cancer spreads.

4. **Use overhead transparency** 10-3 to answer the question, What causes cance? Point out that medical science has learned much about what causes cancer in recent years, but there is still much that is not known. Discuss the cancer risk factors.

5. **Show overhead transparency** 56 (from the color transparency packet) to show the relative role of then major risk factors that cause cancer.

6. **Write on the chalkboard** the following numbers; 33, 18, 15, and 4. Ask the students what the numbers represent (see "What are Your Chances" on the previous page).

7. **Show overhead transparency** 10-4 and discuss the incidence of cancer and the survival rates for various types of cancer. Contrast the rates for men and women.

8. **Show overhead transparency** 10-5 and discuss what can be done to improve one's chances of recovering from cancer. Emphasize the seven danger signals of cancer, the importance of self-examinations, and medical screening procedurtes.

9. **Discuss** specific details about the more frequent cancer sites.

WHAT IS CANCER ?

Cancer is a family of diseases characrterized by abnormal and uncontrolled cell growth.

- **Abnormal cell divilsion**
- **Abnormal chromosome configuration**
- **Abnormal shape and size**
- **Grows and spreads rapaidly**
- **No uweful function**

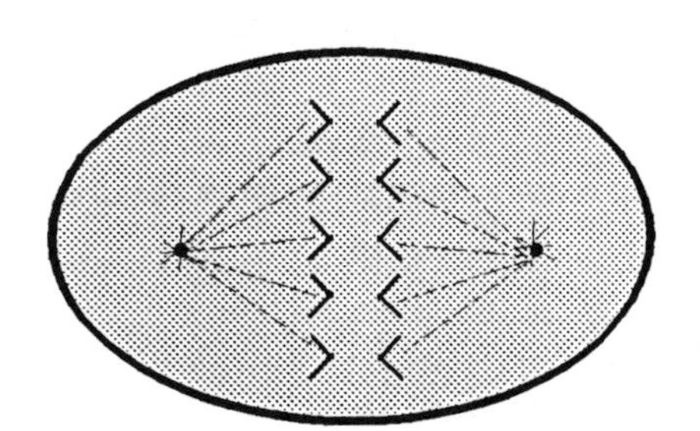

Normal Cell Division

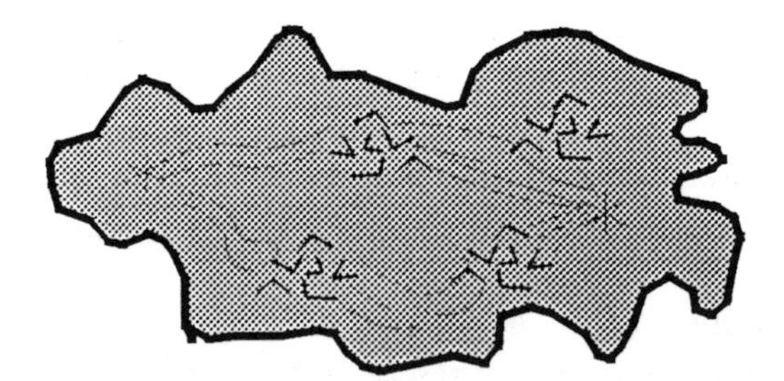

Cancer Cell Division

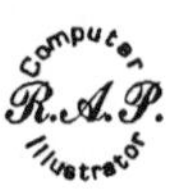

10-1

WHAT IS CANCER ?

Cancer is a type of tumors (neoplasm)
There are two main types of tumors.

1. BENEIGN (non-cancerous tumor)

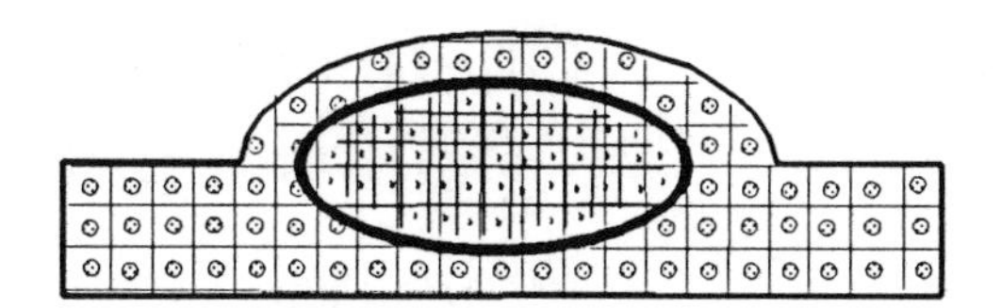

Walled off, May grow,
but does nnot spread.

2. MALIGNANT (cancerous tumor)

Grows and spreads two ways.

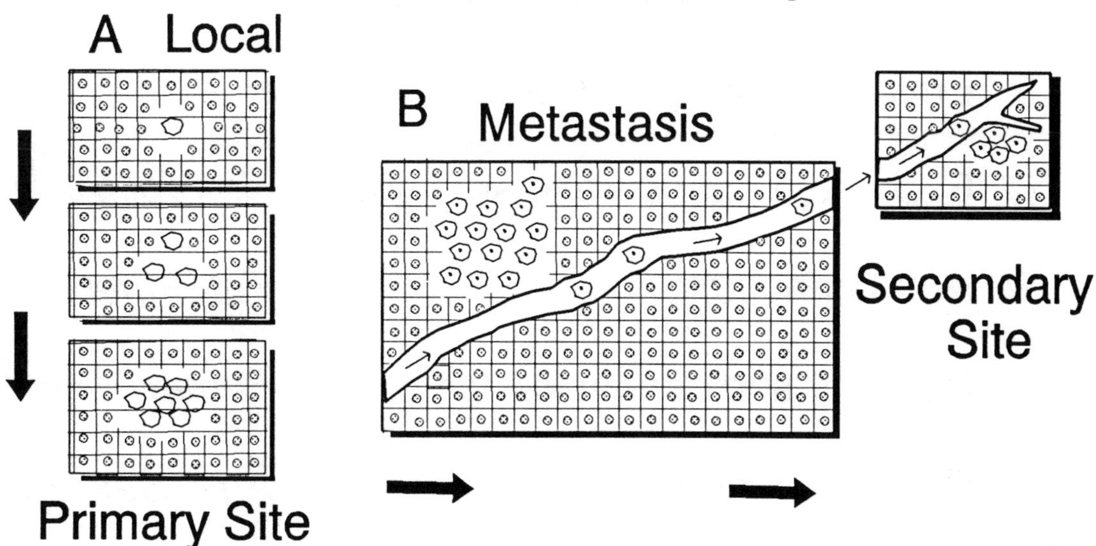

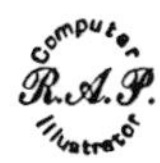

10-2

WHAT CAUSES CANCER 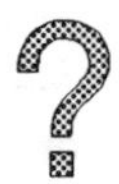

Theories Irritants promote cancer growth.

Irritants

Radiation	Chemical Agents (Carcinogens)
Virusis	Physical Trauma

Risks

- Smoking, smokeless tobacco --- *Smokers, ETS.*
- Environmental pollution ---------- *Public, Work*
- Excessive exposure to sunlight--- *Natural, Artificial*
- Nutritional factors ---------------- *Fat, Fiber*
- Heredity anc congenital factors --- *Family History*
- Personal factors ------------------- *Age, Sex, Race*

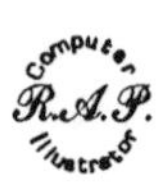

10-3

RECOVERY FROM CANCER:

Improve Your Chances Through EARLY Detection and Treatment

Cancer's Seven Danger Signals

- Hoarseness or Cough
- Change in a Wart or Mole
- A Sore that does not heal
- Unusual bleeding or discharge
- Change in Bowel or Bladder habits
- Indigestion or difficulty swallowing
- A Lump or thickening in the Breast or elsewhere

SELF-EXAMS:

♀ Breast Exam
♂ Testicle Exam

MEDICAL EXAMS:

♀ Paps Test
♂ Prostate Exam
♂♀ Proctoscope

Smear, Biopsy, / Surgery, Radiation, Chemotherapy

AVOID CANCER QUACKERY !

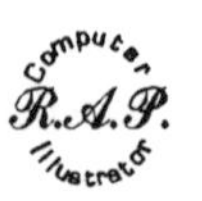

10-5

CANCER STATISTICS

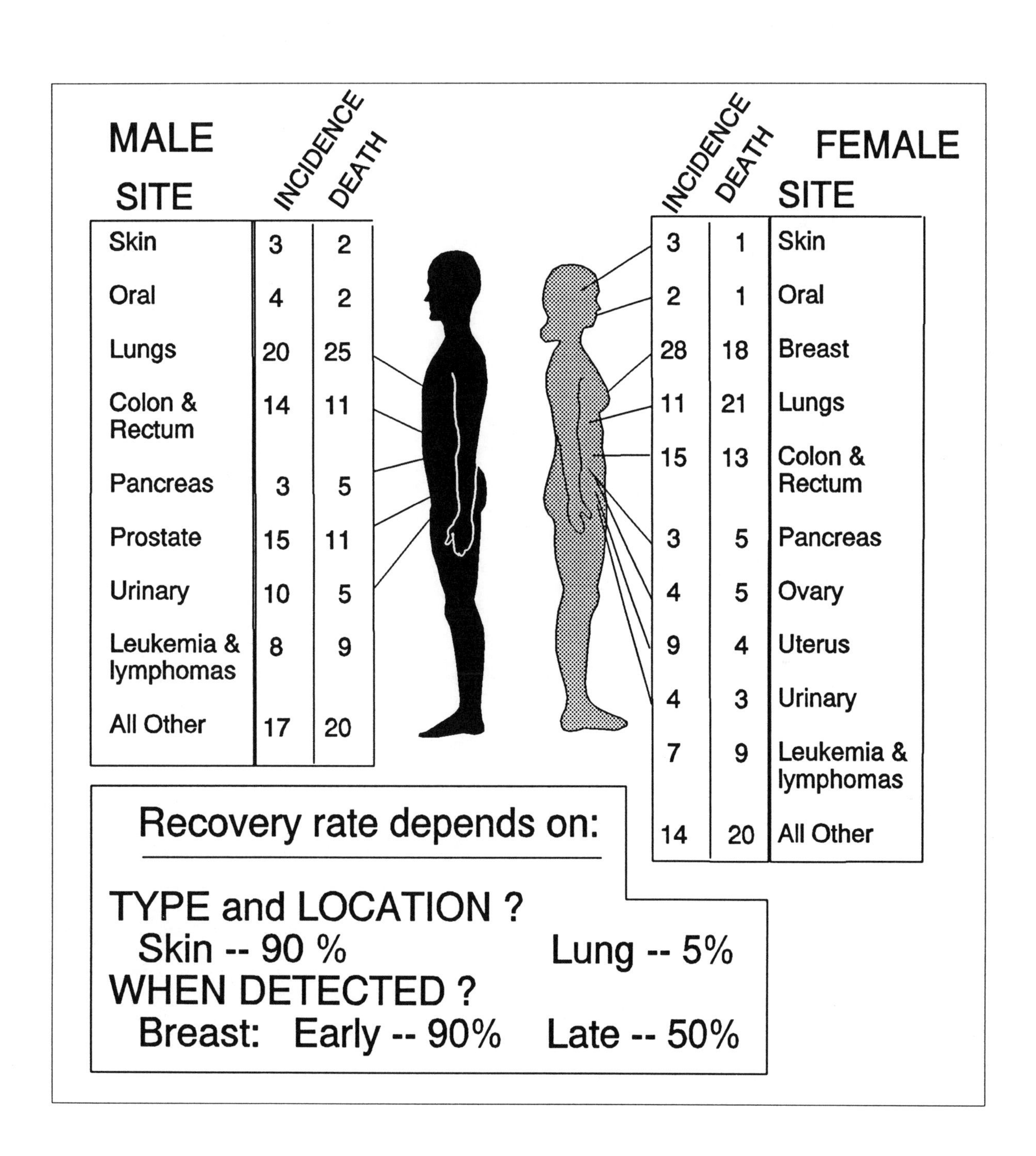

MALE SITE	INCIDENCE	DEATH
Skin	3	2
Oral	4	2
Lungs	20	25
Colon & Rectum	14	11
Pancreas	3	5
Prostate	15	11
Urinary	10	5
Leukemia & lymphomas	8	9
All Other	17	20

INCIDENCE	DEATH	FEMALE SITE
3	1	Skin
2	1	Oral
28	18	Breast
11	21	Lungs
15	13	Colon & Rectum
3	5	Pancreas
4	5	Ovary
9	4	Uterus
4	3	Urinary
7	9	Leukemia & lymphomas
14	20	All Other

Recovery rate depends on:

TYPE and LOCATION ?
Skin -- 90 % Lung -- 5%
WHEN DETECTED ?
Breast: Early -- 90% Late -- 50%

10-4

Stress Assessment and Management Techniques

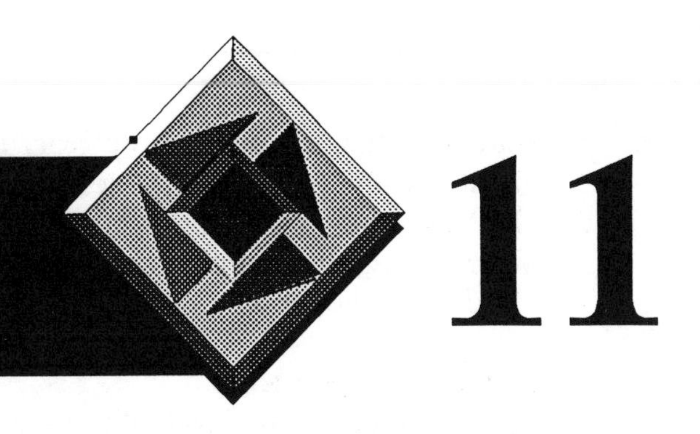

11

Expanded Chapter Outline

I. STRESS

A. Stress is a part of life.

1. The unpredictable changes in modern living are particularly stressful.
2. Stress is one of the most common health problems we face today.
3. Estimates place the cost of stress and stress-related diseases in excess of $100 billion annually in the U.S.:
   a. the cost of treating stress-related diseases produces more stress.
   b. lost productivity and absenteeism on the job cost even more.

B. The good news is that stress can be self-controlled.

1. Most people have learned to accept stress as a normal part of life.
2. Yet, few seem to understand it or know how to cope with it effectively.

C. What is stress?

1. Dr. Hans Selye, a foremost authorities on stress, defined stress as,
   a. *the nonspecific response of the human organism to any demand placed upon it.*
   b. "nonspecific" indicates that the body reacts the same regardless of the nature of the event that leads to the stress.
2. Stress is the body's emotional and physiological response to any situation that is new, threatening, frightening, or exciting.

D. Stress prepares a person to react to the stress-causingevent, or stressor.

1. We do not all react the same way to the same stressor.
2. Our reaction determines whether stress is positive or negative.
   a. many people thrive under stress
   b. others under similar circumstances are unable to handle it
3. The problem is not the stress, but the way we react to stress.

E. **Selye defined the way in which we react to stress as either:**
   1. Eustress--the pleasant or beneficial stress.
   2. Distress--the unpleasant or harmful stress.
   3. In eustress, health and performance continue to improve.
   4. In distress, health and performance begin to deteriorate.

F. **When is stress a problem?**
   1. Everyone needs the level of stress that is conducive to health and adequate performance.
   2. However, when stress reaches certain limits, it keeps the person from functioning effectively.
   3. Chronic distress raises the risk for many health disorders:
      a. coronary heart disease
      b. hypertension
      c. eating disorders
      d. ulcers
      e. diabetes
      f. asthma
      g. depression
      h. migraine headaches
      i. sleep disorders
      j. chronic fatigue
      k. and perhaps even certain types of cancers
   4. Recognizing this turning point and overcoming the problem quickly and efficiently are crucial in maintaining emotional and physiological stability.

II. SOURCES OF STRESS

A. **Several instruments have been developed to assess sources of stress in life.**

B. **One instrument is the Life Experiences Survey (Figure 11.2).**
   1. Identifies life changes that may impact health.
   2. Contains a list of 47 life events.
   3. Also provides for other events not listed in the survey.
   4. You rate the extent the events you experienced had a positive or negative impact on your life at the time of the event.
   5. After scoring each event, a "total life change" score is obtained.
   6. The total life change score is a good indicator of total life stress.

III. BEHAVIOR PATTERNS

A. **The two main types of behavior patterns are Type A and Type B.**
   1. Type A behavior characteristics:
      a. hard-driving

   b. overambitious
   c. aggressive
   d. at times hostile
   e. overly competitive
   f. set their own goals
   g. are self-motivated
   h. try to accomplish many tasks at the same time
   i. excessively achievement-oriented
   j. have a high degree of time urgency
2. Type B behavior characteristics:
   a. calm
   b. casual
   c. relaxed
   d. easy-going
   e. takes one thing at a time
   f. do not feel pressured or hurried
   g. seldom set their own deadlines

B. Researchers found that Type A individualshad a higher incidence of coronary heart disease.
1. Type A is associated with too much stress.
2. Type A individuals were counseled to lower their stress level by modifying many of their Type A behaviors.
3. Many Type A characteristics are learned behaviors that can be modified to help a person become more Type B.
4. However, a debate centered on which Type A behaviors should be changed.

C. New evidence indicates that not all typical Type A people are at higher risk.
1. Now, only certain characteristics put one at higher risk:
   a. anger
   b. hostility
2. Many behavioral modification counselors work on changing these behaviors.

D. More recently, the term Type C has been used to describe individualswho as highly stressed as Type A's, but have no higher risk than Type B's.
1. The keys to successful Type C performance seem to be:
   a. commitment
   b. confidence
   c. control
2. Type C people are:
   a. highly committed to what they are doing
   b. have a great deal of confidence in their ability to do their work
   c. are in constant control of their actions
3. In addition, they enjoy their work and maintain themselves in top physical condition to be able to meet the mental and physical demands of their work.

E. **Type A behavior by itself is no longer viewed as a major risk factor for coronary heart disease.**
   1. Those especially vulnerable are those who are impatient and readily annoyed when they have to wait for someone or something:
      a. an employee
      b. a traffic light
      c. a restaurant line
   2. Counseling is focusing on individuals who:
      a. have anxiety
      b. have depression
      c. have feelings of helplessness
      d. lose control of their lives
      e. give up on their dreams in life

IV. VULNERABILITY TO STRESS

A. **A number of factors affect the way we handle stress.**

B. **The questionnaire provided in Figure 11.3 lists these factors.**
   1. Many of the items on this questionnaire are related to:
      a. health
      b. social support
      c. self-worth
      d. nurturance (sense of being needed)
   2. The questionnaire will help you identify specific areas of needed improvement.
   3. How people deal with these factors can increase or decrease vulnerability to stress.

C. **All of the factors are crucial for a person's health and wellbeing.**
   1. The benefits of physical fitness is emphasized in this book.
   2. Social, mental, and emotional well-being is are discussed extensively.

D. **Positive correlations have been found between social support and health outcomes.**
   1. People can draw upon social support to weather crises.
   2. Knowing that someone cares and that support is out there is valuable in times of need.

E. **Strength comes when we realize that many factors influencing stress are under our own control.**
   1. People can improve behaviors that make them more vulnerable to stress.
   2. Start by modifying the behaviors that are easiest to change.

F. **Nurturance is another factor that affects the way people handle stress.**
   1. People who make the effort to help others end up helping themselves even more.
   2. We benefit emotionally from the sense of being needed.

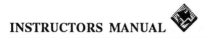

V. TIME MANAGEMENT

A. The present "hurry-up" style of life is not conducive to wellness.

1. People who do not manage their time properly will quickly experience:
   a. chronic stress
   b. fatigue, despair
   c. discouragement
   d. illness
2. In one poll, almost half of the respondents wished they had more time for exercise, recreation, hobbies, and family.
3. Healthy and successful people are good time managers:
   a. Harvard graduates attributed their success to *smart work*, not *hard work*
   b. the most successful rated himself as a superior time manager

B. Five Steps to Time Management:

1. Find out how you spend each part of the day:
   a. keep a log for a week
   b. record your activities at half-hour intervals
   c. at the end of each day, decide when you wasted time
   d. common time killers are:
      (1) watching television
      (2) listening to radio/music
      (3) sleeping
      (4) eating
      (5) daydreaming
      (6) shopping
      (7) socializing/parties
      (8) recreation
      (9) talking on the telephone
      (10) worrying
      (11) procrastination
      (12) drop-in visitors
      (13) confusion (unclear goals)
      (14) indecision (what to do next)
      (15) interruptions
      (16) perfectionism (every detail must be done)
   e. some of these activities are necessary, but in excess they'll lead to stress in life.
2. Set long-range and short-range goals:
   a. this requires some in-depth thinking to put your life in perspective.
      (1) what do I want out of life?
      (2) where do I want to be in 10 years? Next year? Next week? Tomorrow?
3. Identify your immediate goals, and prioritize them for today and this week.
   a. each day determine what you need to accomplish that day, and that week.
   b. rank your "today" and "this week" tasks in four categories:

      (1) top-priority--most important
      (2) medium-priority--must be done but can wait
      (3) low-priority,--to be done after top and medium tasks are done
      (4) "trash."-- not worth your time

4. Use a daily planner to help you organize and simplify your day:
   a. as you plan your day, be realistic
   b. recognize your most productive time for work, study, errands
   c. pick your best hours for top-priority activities
   d. be sure to schedule enough time for exercise and relaxation
5. Take 10 minutes each night to evaluate yourself daily.
   a. cross off the goals you accomplished
   b. carry over to the next day those you did not get done
   c. you also may realize that some goals can be moved down to low-priority
   d. others can be trashed

C. **Time-Management Skills:**
   1. The following can help you make better use of your time:
      a. delegate
      b. say "no"
      c. protect against boredom
      d. plan ahead for disruptions
      e. get it done
      f. eliminate distractions
      g. set aside "overtimes" for under scheduled projects
      h. plan time for you
      i. reward yourself

VI. COPING WITH STRESS

A. **Stress is a problem when it interferes with optimal level of health and performance.**

B. **The way people perceive and cope with stress is more important than the stress itself.**

C. **Several stress management techniques can help people cope more effectively:**
   1. First, the person must recognize that a problem exists:
      a. many people do not want to believe they are under too much stress
      b. many people fail to recognize some of the typical symptoms of distress
      c. noting some of the stress-related symptoms might help
   2. Second, try to identify the stress-related symptoms and remove the stressor.
      a. removing the stress-causing agent is not simple
      b. in some situations eliminating the stressor is not know
      c. in many instances the stressor cannot be removed
   3. When the stressor cannot be identified, keeping a log of when symptoms occur and events preceding the symptoms may help identify the stressor.

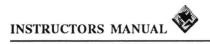

4. When the stressor can't be removed the stress can be managed through relaxation techniques.

D. The body responds to stress by activating the fight-or-flight mechanism.

1. This prepares a person to take action by stimulating the body's defense systems.
2. This stimulation originates in the hypothalamus and the pituitary gland.
3. The hypothalamus activates the sympathetic nervous system.
4. The pituitary activates the release of catecholamines (hormones) from the adrenal glands.
5. These hormonal changes increase:
   a. heart rate
   b. blood pressure
   c. blood flow to active muscles and the brain
   d. glucose levels
   e. oxygen consumption
   f. strength
6. After the fight or flight response, the body relaxes and stress dissipates.
7. But if the person is unable to take action, the body changes continue.
8. This increased tension and tightening can be dissipated effectively through some coping techniques.

VII. RELAXATION TECHNIQUES

A. The following relaxation techniques may be helpful in managing stress:

1. Some benefits of relaxation may be realized almost immediately.
2. The full benefits may not be gained until after months of regular practice.
3. If these exercises are not effective, professional help may be called for.

B. Biofeedback:

1. Has become a popular treatment for a variety of medical disorders.
   a. become an effective technique for managing:
      (1) stress
      (2) essential hypertension
      (3) asthma
      (4) heart rhythm rate disturbances
      (5) cardiac neurosis
      (6) eczematous dermatitis
      (7) fecal incontinence
      (8) insomnia
      (9) stuttering
2. Biofeedback as a treatment modality has been defined as:
   a. a process in which a person learns to reliably influence two kinds of physiological responses:
      (1) responses which are not ordinarily under voluntary control

(2) responses ordinarily under voluntary control, but for which regulation has broken down due to trauma or disease.

b. in biofeedback the person can "feel" how thought processes influence biological responses:

(1) heart rate
(2) blood pressure
(3) body temperature
(4) muscle tension

3. Some biofeedback instruments are simple but most are complex.
   a. requires expensive complex electronic instruments
   b. also requires adequately trained personnel
   c. teaches people how to influence physiological responses
   d. entails a three-stage, closed-loop feedback system:
      (1) a biological response to a stressor is detected and amplified
      (2) the response is processed
      (3) results of the response are fed back to the individual immediately
4. Physical exercise and progressive muscle relaxation have been used successfully as an alternative to biofeedback in stress management.

C. **Physical Activity:**

1. Physical activity is one of the simplest tools to control stress.
2. The value of exercise in reducing stress is related to several factors.
   a. decreases muscular tension.
   b. helps to metabolize the increased catecholamines associated with the fight-or-flight mechanism.
   c. the early evening hours in a health club are becoming the most popular time and place to exercise for a lot of highly stressed executives.
   d. helps them dissipate the stress accumulated during the day.
   e. although exercise does not solve problems, it can help a person cope with stress, preventing it from becoming a chronic problem.
3. Physical exercise that is vigorous, continuous, and rhythmic works well.
   a. it stimulates the same alpha-wave activity in the brain as does meditation and relaxation
   b. morphine-like substances (endorphines) are thought to be released from the pituitary gland in the brain
   c. these substances not only act as painkillers but also seem to induce a soothing and calming effect
   d. physical exercise gives people a psychological boost because it:
      (1) lessens feelings of anxiety, depression, frustration, aggression, anger, and hostility
      (2) alleviates insomnia
      (3) provides an opportunity to meet social needs
      (4) allows the person to share common interests and problems
      (5) develops discipline
4. Exercise provides the opportunity to do something enjoyable and constructive that

will lead to better health and total well-being.

a. the cardiovascular system is affected seriously by stress
b. aerobic exercise not only strengthens the cardiovascular system, it also helps a person cope more effectively with the effects of stress
c. fit individuals can cope more effectively and are less affected by the stresses of daily living

D. **Progressive Relaxation—you contract, then relax the muscles of the body.**

1. Lie on your back in the most comfortable position possible. Loosen any restrictive clothing. Close your eyes, rotate your ankles outward, and put your arms at your sides.
2. Starting with your feet, involve all major muscle groups in the body. Don't forget your face, including your forehead, eyes, nose, mouth, cheeks, and tongue.
3. As you move to each muscle group, contract the muscles as tightly as you can and hold the contraction for 20 or 30 seconds, then relax.
4. Concentrate on the dramatic difference in feeling between a tensed muscle and a relaxed one. With practice, you'll be able to achieve relaxation "on demand."

E. **Breathing Techniques—breathing exercises can be learned in only a few minutes.**

1. Sit in a comfortable position with hands folded over your abdomen, just over your navel.
2. Keeping your eyes open, imagine a balloon lying beneath your hands.
3. Begin to slowly inhale through your nose, concentrating on the warm air entering your nose and slowly filling the balloon.
4. When the balloon is full (this should take 3 to 4 seconds initially), slowly exhale to empty the balloon, feeling your chest and abdomen relaxing.
5. Repeat the entire process two or three times. Each time concentrate on "breathing away" the tension and inhaling fresh oxygen.
6. When finished, sit quietly for a few minutes before rising.

F. **Autogenic—similar to progressive relaxation, followed by imagery that extends the relaxed state.**

1. Sit in a straight back chair in a quiet room with mild temperature, free of distractions.
2. Assume the most comfortable position with your feet flat on the floor, your head hanging loosely forward, your eyes closed, and your hands in your lap with your palms turned upward. Loosen any restrictive clothing.
3. Imagine the parts of your body are tired, heavy, and warm like just after a strenuous workout. Begin with your legs. As you inhale and exhale deeply and slowly, repeat "My legs are so tired. My legs are so heavy. My legs are very heavy and warm."
4. Move to other muscle groups—buttocks, abdomen, chest, arms, shoulders, and so on. You even might imagine your internal organs, such as your stomach and your heart, relaxed and warm.
5. Concentrate on how cool your forehead feels. For you to feel refreshed and alert,

your forehead must feel cool.

6. Once your entire body is relaxed, visualize an image you find relaxing. It might be waves lapping against a sandy beach, a cloud drifting lazily across the afternoon sky, an eagle soaring silently. The image should lead you to total relaxation.

G. **Meditation is a mental exercise that can bring about psychological benefits.**
   1. The objective of meditation is to gain control over one's attention.
   2. It clears the mind and blocks out the stressor(s).
   3. This technique can be learned rather quickly.
   4. It can be used frequently during times of increased tension and stress.
   5. Initially the person who is learning to meditate should:
      a. Choose a room that is comfortable, quiet, and free of disturbances.
      b. After learning the technique, it can be done almost anywhere.
      c. It requires a time block of approximately 15 minutes, twice a day.
   6. The process is as follows:
      a. Sit in a chair in an upright position with the hands resting either in your lap or on the arms of the chair.
      b. Close your eyes and focus on your breathing.
      c. Allow your body to relax, assume a passive attitude.
      d. Concentrate on your breathing.
         (1) allow the body to breathe regularly, at its own rhythm.
         (2) repeat in your mind, the word "one" as you inhale.
         (3) repeat the word "two" every time you exhale. (This is done to keep distressing thoughts from entering into your mind.)
         (4) continue to breathe in this way for about 15 minutes.
         (5) this time has been set aside for meditation, and you need to relax, take your time, and enjoy the exercise.

VIII. WHICH TECHNIQUE IS BEST?

A. **Each person reacts to stress differently.**

B. **The best coping strategy is one which works.**

C. **You may want to experiment with all of them to find out which works best.**

D. **A combination of two or more works best for many people.**

E. **People need to learn to relax and take time out for themselves.**

F. **The time spent doing stress management exercises (several times a day, as needed) is well worth the effort if stress is a significant problem.**

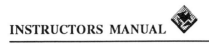

Instructor Activities

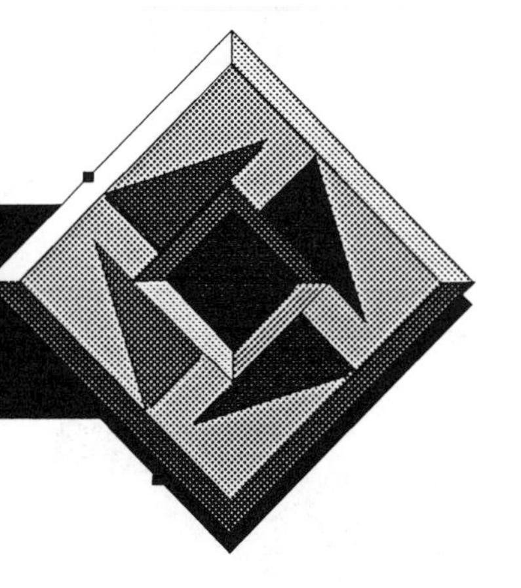

1. **Use overhead transparency 11-1** (master found in this manual) to explain what stress is. Help the students better understand the role of stress as it relates to wellness. Follow the expanded outline Section I and II.

2. **Use overhead transparency 11-2** (master found in this manual) and discuss the function of homeostasis.

3. **Use overhead transparency 11-3** (master found in this manual) and discuss the stages of General Adaptation Syndrome (GAS). Follow the expanded outline Section I part D.

4. **Use color overhead transparency 58** (found color packet) to discuss the relationship between stress and health and performance. Eustress enables an individual to perform at an optimal level.

4. **Use color overhead transparency 59** (found in the color packet) to discuss the physiological response to stress. Follow the expanded outline Section I part D.

5. **Use overhead transparency 11-4** (master found in this manual) to show how an appropriate amount of stress can be beneficial in dealing with emergencies, but that chronic stress can cause illness. Stress can be beneficial if the emergency chemicals produced by stress can be used in appropriate physical activity which will effectively resolve the situation. However, if the emergency chemicals are not used, through some physical activity, they accumulate in the body, disrupt homeostasis, and cause injury to vulnerable organs. Also distinguish between eustress and distress. Point out that too much eustress can also be harmful. Follow the expanded outline Section I parts E and F.

6. **Use overhead transparency 11-5** (master found in this manual) in a discussion about coping with stress. Point out that carrying a cellular phone in a golf bag might not be an effective strategy for relaxation. Talk about sources of help where one can go to learn relaxation techniques, make use of biofeedback, network, and get counseling.

WHAT IS STRESS?

Stress is the body's **biochemicalresponse**
to
perceiveddemands.

STRESSOR

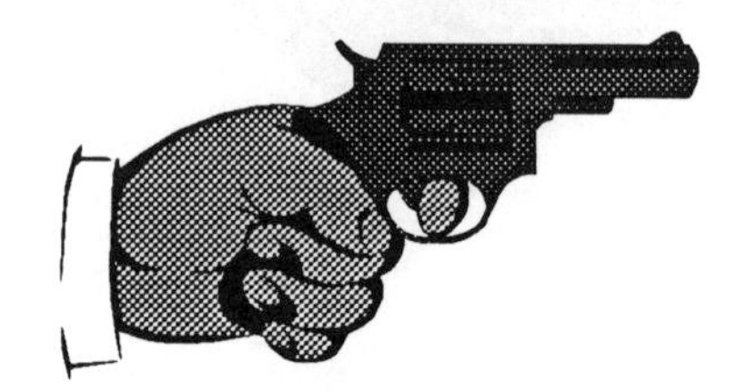

real or imagined
current or future
intrinsic or extrinsic
pleasant or unpleasant
(eustress or distress)

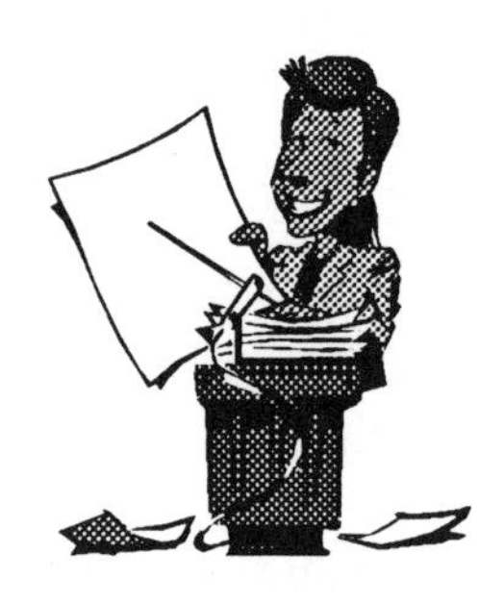
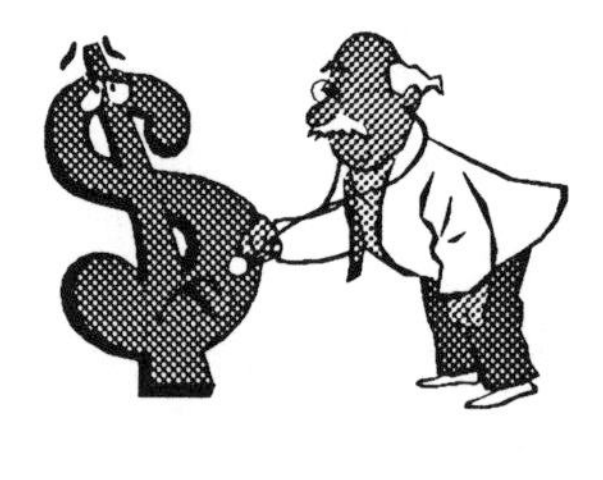
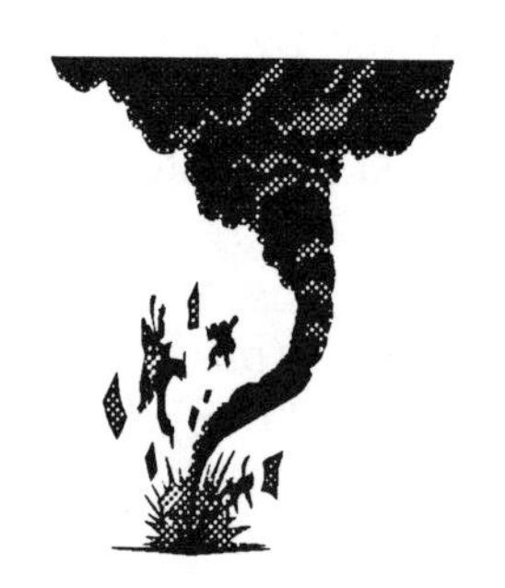
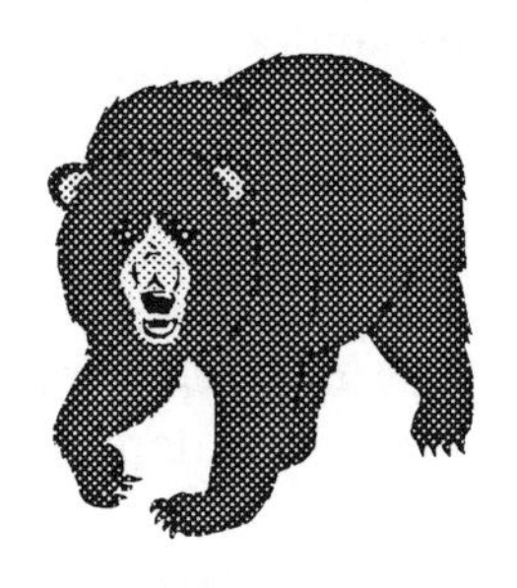

EMOTIONALAND PHYSIOLOGICALRESPONSE
Stress prepares a person to react to the stress-causing event, or stressor.

Nervous System -- sympathetic or parasympathetic
Endocrine System -- emergency harmonies

11-1

⁰ What is Homeostasis?

HOMEOSTASIS

The body has a tendency to maintain an equilibrium or consistent balance in it's *physiological* functions.

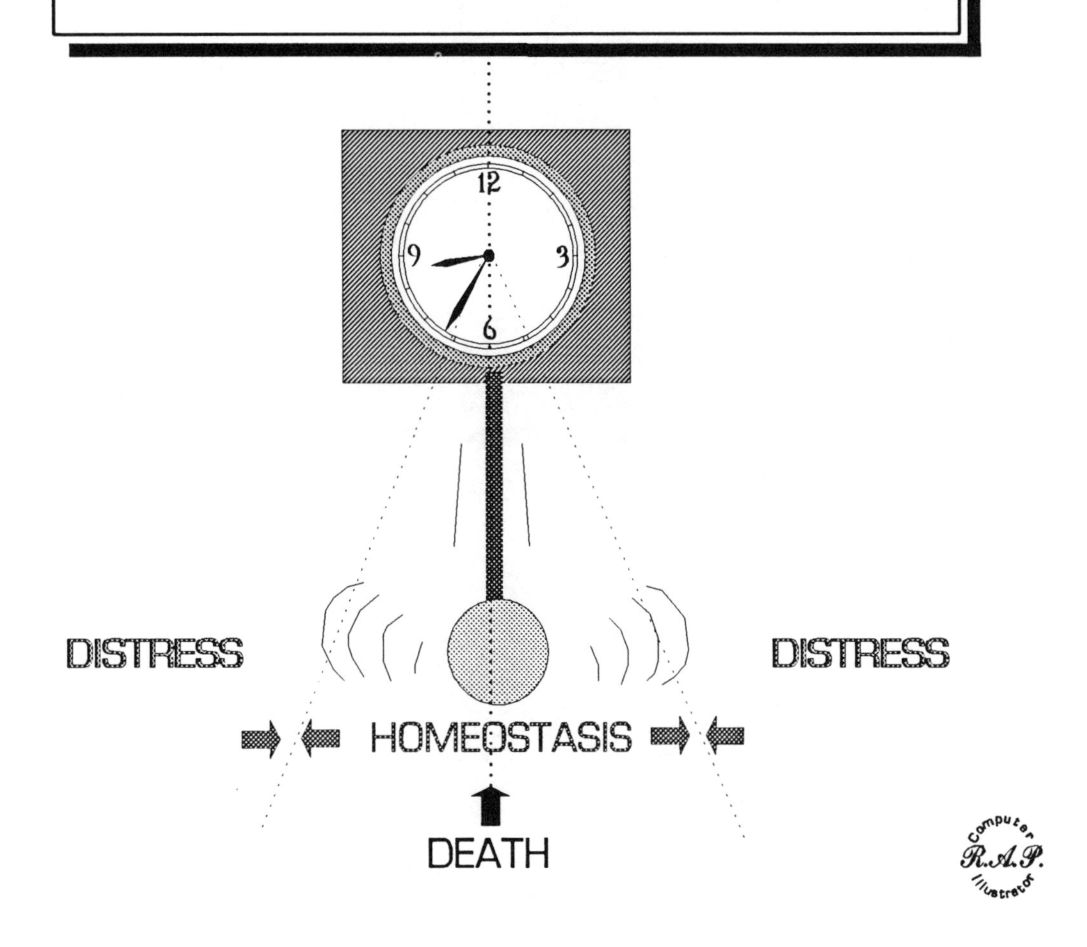

11-2

The Stress Response GSA

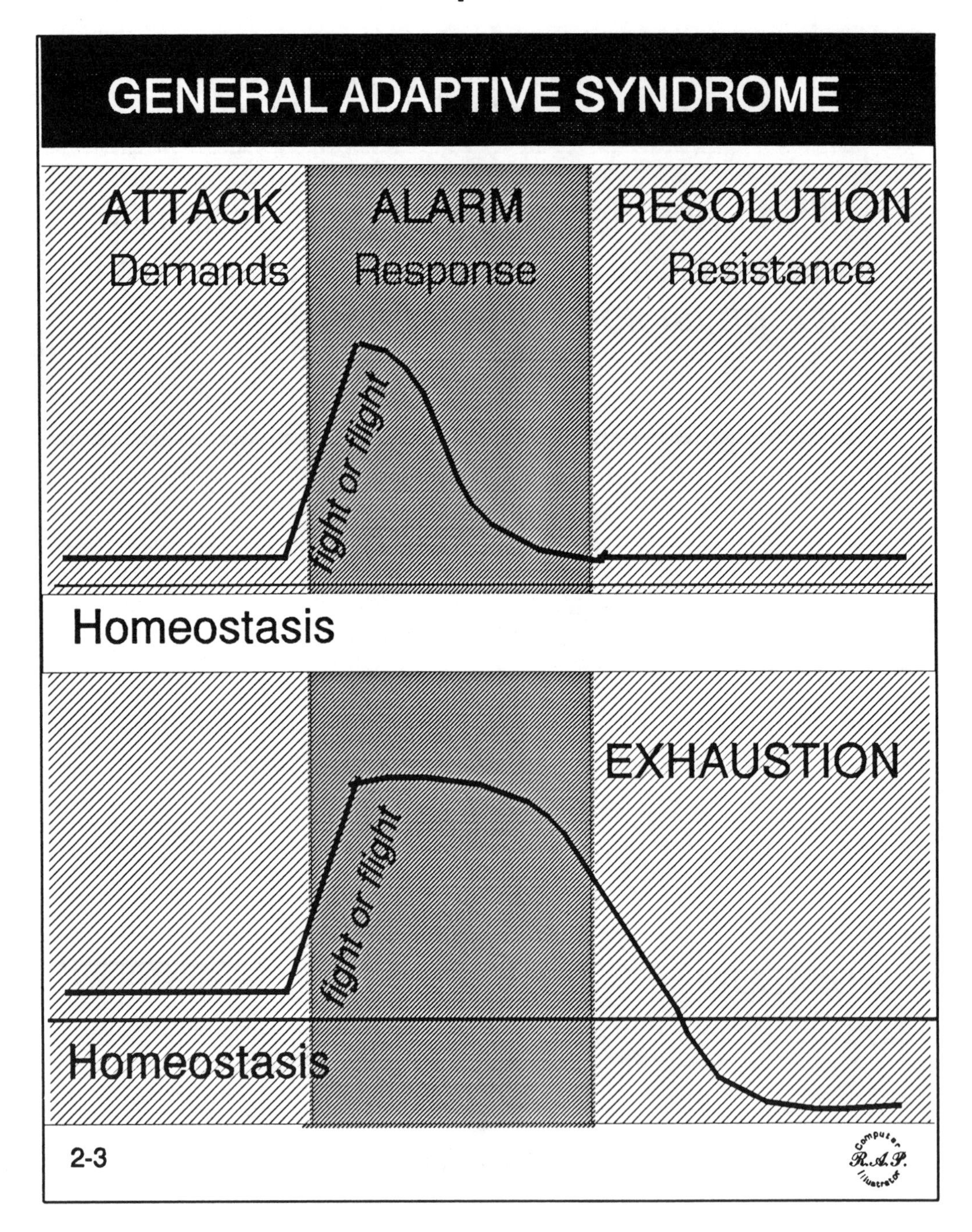

11-3

The Stress Theory Selye

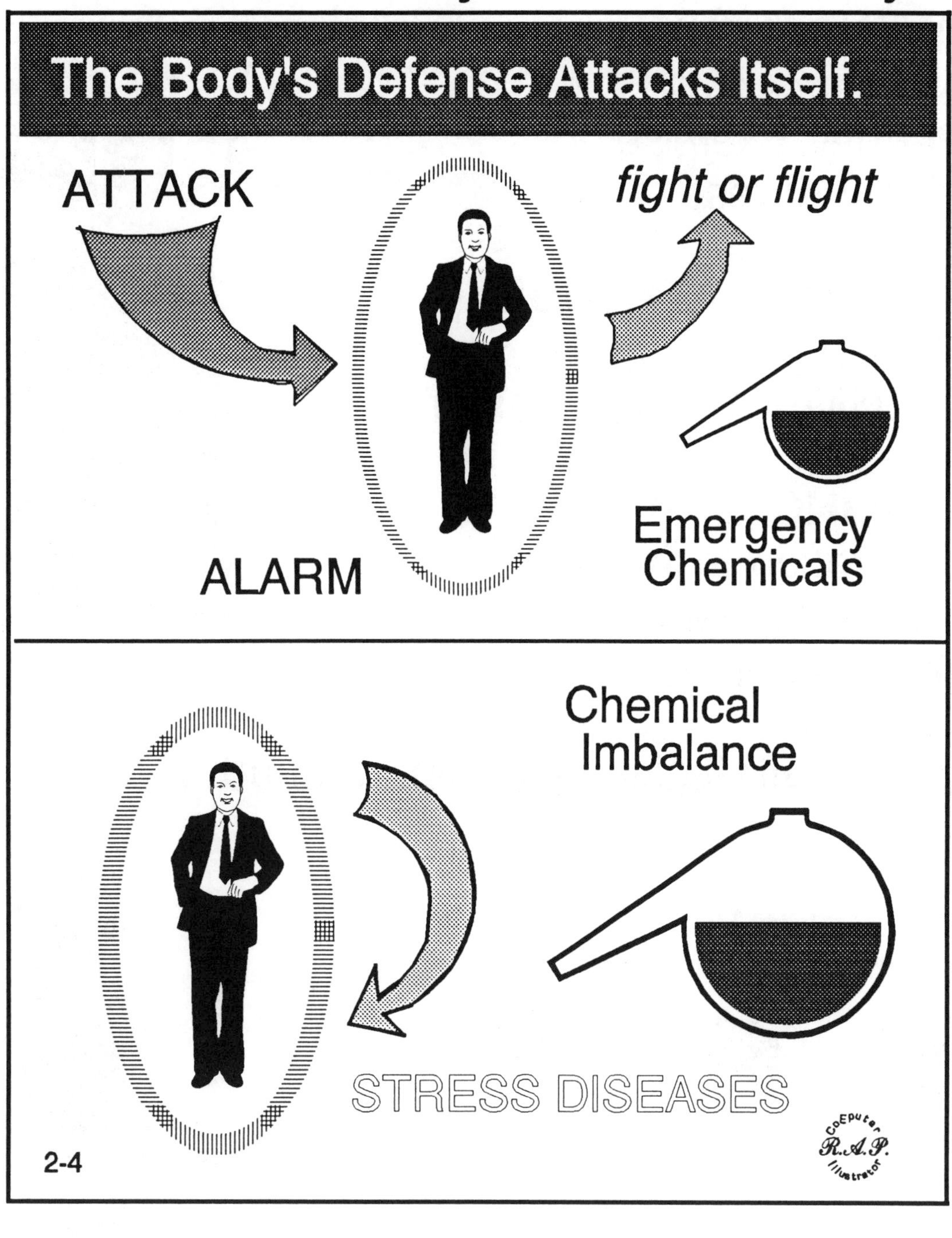

11-4

COPING WITH STRESS

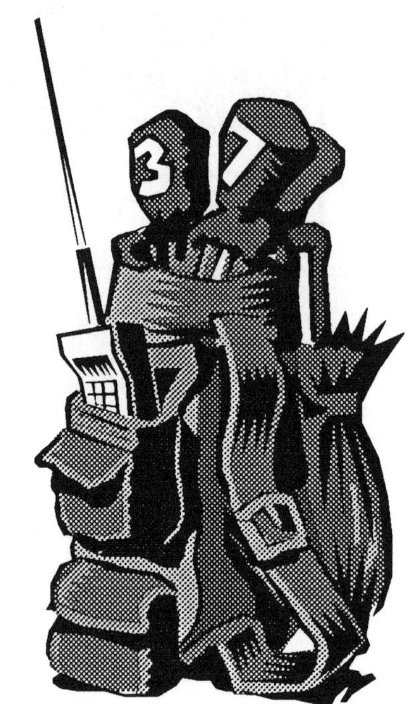

STAY HEALTHY

A balanced diet
Regular Exercise
Plenty of rest

A POSITIVE ATTITUDE

Refreshing thoughts
Effective time management

HANDLING STRESS

Relaxation techniques
Burnout prevention
Social support
Laughter
(Select strategies that help, not hurt.

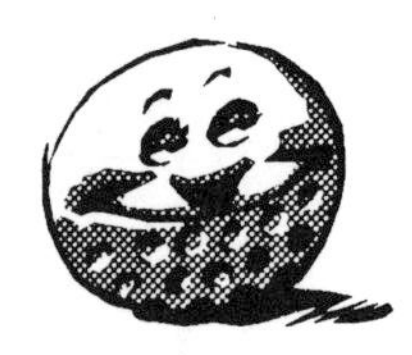

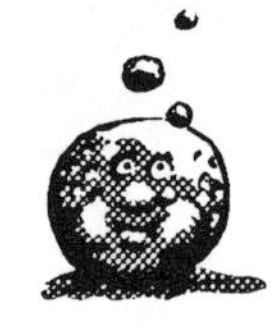

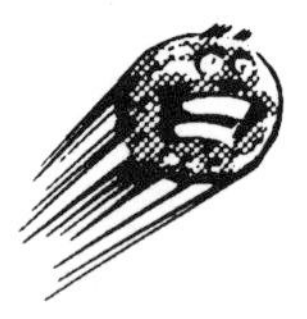

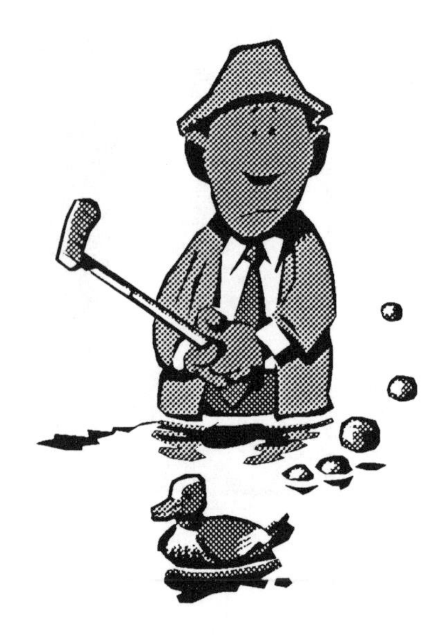

11-5

Introduction to Lifetime Physical Fitness and Wellness

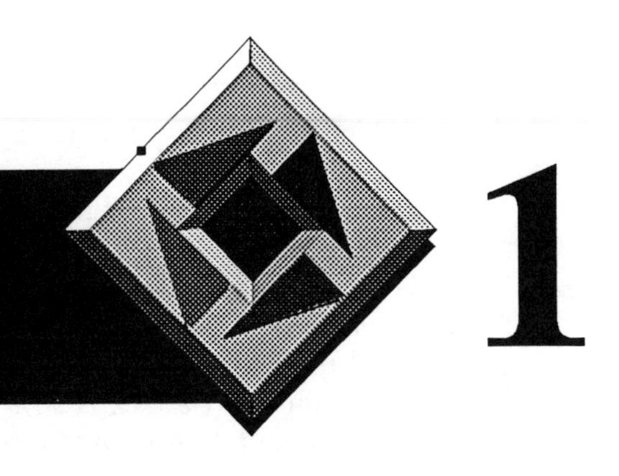

1

Expanded Chapter Outline

I. TOBACCO

A. Tobacco has been smoked throughout the world for hundreds of years.
1. Before 1800 it was used primarily in the form of pipes or cigars.
2. Cigarette smoking did not become popular until the mid-1800s.
3. Smoking increased dramatically at the turn of the century.

B. The harmful effects of tobacco use were not well known until the early 1960s.
1. U.S. Surgeon General issued the first major report in 1964.
2. Tobacco use in all its forms is now a significant threat to life.
3. 10% of all people will die as a result of smoking-related illnesses.

II. CIGARETTE SMOKING

A. Cigarette smoking is the largest preventable cause of illness and premature death in the United States:
1. Smoking is responsible for more than 450,000 deaths each year.
2. These deaths are all unnecessary.
3. Smoking increases the death rates from:
   a. heart disease
   b. cancer
   c. stroke
   d. aortic aneurysm
   e. chronic bronchitis
   f. emphysema
   g. peptic ulcers
4. Cigarette smoking by pregnant women has been linked to:
   a. retarded fetal growth

    b. higher risk for spontaneous abortion
    c. prenatal death
5. Smoking also is the most prevalent cause of injury and death from fire.

B. The average life expectancy for a chronic smoker is as much as 18 years shorter than for a nonsmoker.

1. A 1993 report indicated that each cigarette shortens life by 7 minutes.
2. The risk for heart attack is 50% to 100% higher for smokers.
3. The mortality rate following heart attacks also is higher for smokers.

C. Cigarette smoking affects the cardiovascular system.

1. Smoking increases:
    a. heart rate
    b. blood pressure
    c. susceptibility to atherosclerosis
    d. potential for blood clots
2. Smoking decreases:
    a. high-density lipoprotein (HDL) cholesterol
    b. oxygen carrying capacity of the blood.

D. Tobacco increases the risk of cancer.

1. 83% of lung cancer and 30% of all cancers are attributable to smoking.
2. Tobacco use increases the risk for cancer of the:
    a. oral cavity
    b. larynx
    c. esophagus
    d. bladder
    e. pancreas
    f. kidneys
    g. lung
3. Although half of all cancers are curable, the 5-year survival rate for lung cancer is less than 13%.
4. Tobacco kills about 142,000 people each year.

E. There is an economic impact of cigarette smoking.

1. American business and industry pays more than $16 billion each year as a direct result of smoking in the workplace.
2. They also pay another $37 billion in lost productivity because of illness, disability, and death.
3. The estimated cost to business for health care each year is between $624 and $4,611 per smoking employee.

F. Nearly 450,000 American die each year because of smoking.

G. What would the public say if that number of people were to die from:

1. airplane accidents
2. a meaningless war
3. a single nonprescription drug

H. Why is there not a greater campaign being waged against tobacco use?
1. Tobacco is the sixth largest cash crop in the United.
2. It produces 2.5% of the gross national product.
3. One tobacco company donated $17 million to organizations such as United Way, YMCA, Salvation Army, Red Cross, etc.

III. SMOKELESS TOBACCO

A. According to the Advisory Committee to the U. S. Surgeon General, smokeless tobacco represents a significanthealth risk.
1. It is not a safe alternative to cigarette smoking.
2. It is just as addictive as cigarette smoking.
3. The use of smokeless tobacco has increased during the last 15 years.
4. The greatest concern is the increase in use by young people.

B. Spit tobacco contains 2.5 times as much nicotine as a pack of cigarettes.
1. Using smokeless tobacco leads to:
   a. gingivitis
   b. periodontitis
   c. oral cancer
   d. premature death
2. People who chew or dip also have:
   a. a higher rate of cavities, sore gums
   b. bad breath
   c. stained teeth
   d. reduced smell or taste
   e. changes in heart rate and blood pressure
   f. increased risk for diseases of the cardiovascular system

C. Using tobacco in any form is addictive and poses a serious threat to health and well-being.

IV. WHY DO PEOPLE SMOKE?

A. People start to smoke for many different reasons, the three most common are:
1. peer pressure,
2. the desire to appear "grown up,"
3. rebellion against authority.

B. People typically begin to smoke without realizing its detrimental effects.

1. Smoking only three packs of cigarettes is enough to cause addiction.
2. Smoking is the most widespread example of drug dependency.

C. More than 1,200 toxic chemicals have been found in tobacco smoke.

1. Nicotine has strong addictive properties.
2. Within seconds, nicotine affects the central nervous system.
3. It can act simultaneously as a tranquilizer and a stimulant.
4. Tar contains about 30 chemical compounds that are proven carcinogens, or cancer-producing agents.

D. People smoke to relax, for pleasure, and as a part or associated activities.

1. Typical associated activities are:
   a. coffee drinking
   b. alcohol drinking
   c. social gatherings
   d. after a meal
   e. talking on the telephone
   f. driving
   g. reading
   h. watching television
2. In many cases the social rituals of smoking are difficult to eliminate.
3. Even years after stopping, people still may crave cigarettes.
4. Most people smoke for a variety of reasons:
   a. stimulation, it wakes you up and keeps you going
   b. handling things can be satisfying
   c. accentuation of pleasure of relaxation
   d. reduction of negative feelings, or "crutch"
   e. craving or dependence
   f. habit

V. SMOKING CESSATION

A. Quitting cigarette smoking is not easy:

1. Only about 20% of smokers who try to quit the first time succeed.
2. The addictive properties of nicotine and smoke make quitting difficult.
3. Some authorities have indicated that nicotine is perhaps the most addictive drug known to humans.
4. Smokers develop a tolerance to nicotine and smoke.
5. They develop both physical and psychological withdrawal symptoms when they stop smoking.

B. Even though giving up smoking can be extremely difficult, it is by no means impossible.

1. More than 95% of successful ex-smokers have been able quit on their own:
   a. some by quitting cold turkey

b. others use self-help kits.

VI. BREAKING THE HABIT

A. The following seven-step plan has helped many people stop smoking in 4 weeks.

1. Step One--Decide positively that you want to quit.
2. Step Two--Begin a personal diet and exercise program:
   a. about one-third of the people who quit smoking gain weight
   b. food may becomes a substitute for cigarettes
   c. appetite increases
   d. basal metabolism may slow down
3. Step Three--Decide on the approach you will use to stop smoking.
   a. cold turkey
   b. gradually
4. Step Four--Keep a daily log of your smoking habit for a few days.
5. Step Five--Set the target date for quitting.
6. Step Six--Stock up on low-calorie foods and drink plenty of water.
7. Step Seven--Do not keep cigarettes handy, stay away from friends who smoke.

B. Replace the old behavior with new behavior:

1. Drink large amounts of water and fruit juices.
2. Talk to someone else.
3. Washing your hands.
4. Brushing your teeth.
5. Eating a healthy snack.
6. Chewing on a straw.
7. Doing dishes.
8. Playing sports.
9. Going for a walk or bike ride.
10. Going swimming.
11. Engage in activities that require the use of your hands.
12. Try gardening, sewing, writing letters, drawing, doing household chores, or washing the car.
13. Visit non-smoking places such as libraries.
14. Plan an outing or a trip away from home.

VII. LIFE AFTER CIGARETTES

A. When you first quit smoking, you can expect a series of withdrawal symptoms:

1. The physiological addiction to nicotine is broken in only 3 days.
2. The first few days may not be as difficult as the first few months.
3. Any of the activities associated with smoking may trigger a relapse even months, or at times years, after quitting.

B. It is never too late to quit.

1. Even though some harm may have been done already, the risk for illness starts to decrease the moment you stop smoking.
2. You will have fewer sore throats and sores in the mouth, less hoarseness, no more cigarette cough, and less risk for peptic ulcers.
3. Circulation to the hands and feet will improve, as will gastrointestinal and kidney and bladder functions.
4. Everything will taste and smell better.
5. You will have more energy, and you will gain a sense of freedom, pride, and well-being.
6. You no longer will have to worry whether you have enough cigarettes to last you through a day, a party, a meeting, a weekend, a trip.

C. Events can trigger your urge to smoke.

1. Avoid rationalizations such as:
   a. "one cigarette won't hurt
   b. I've been off for months (years in some cases)"
   c. "I can handle it. I'll smoke just today"
2. If you do, you will be back to the regular nasty habit.
3. Be prepared to take action in those situations.

D. Start thinking of yourself as a nonsmoker--no "buts" about it.

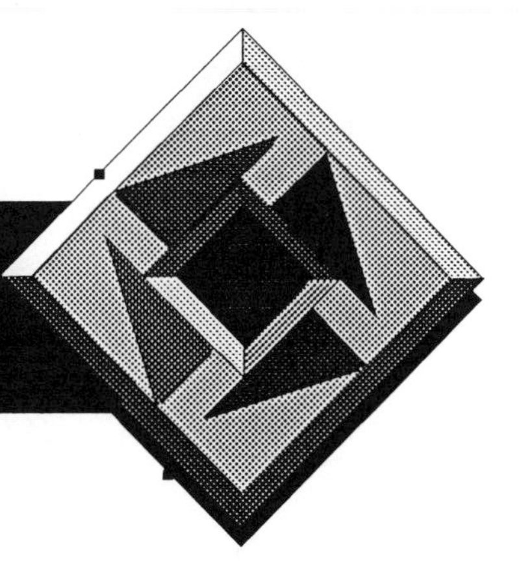

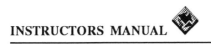

Instructor Activities

1. **Show overhead transparency** 12-1 in this manual to start the discussion about the health problems associated with the uses of tobacco.

2. **Show overhead transparency** 12-2 to discuss the significance of tobacco products as a major health risk.

3. **Show overhead transparency** 12-3 to discuss the effects of tobacco on the heart and vascular system.

4. **Show overhead transparency** 12-4 to discuss the relationship between tobacco and various forms of cancer.

5. **Show overhead transparency** 12-5 to discuss some other effects of smoking and using smokeless tobacco. Emphasize that there are many other health and social problems not mentioned here.

6. **Ask the class** to comment on the current movement to reduce the effects of environmental tobacco smoke in public places and in the working environment.

7. **Show overhead transparency** 12-6 to discuss smoking cessation programs. Anyone who can help others to stop using tobacco would be providing a difficult, but very valuable service.

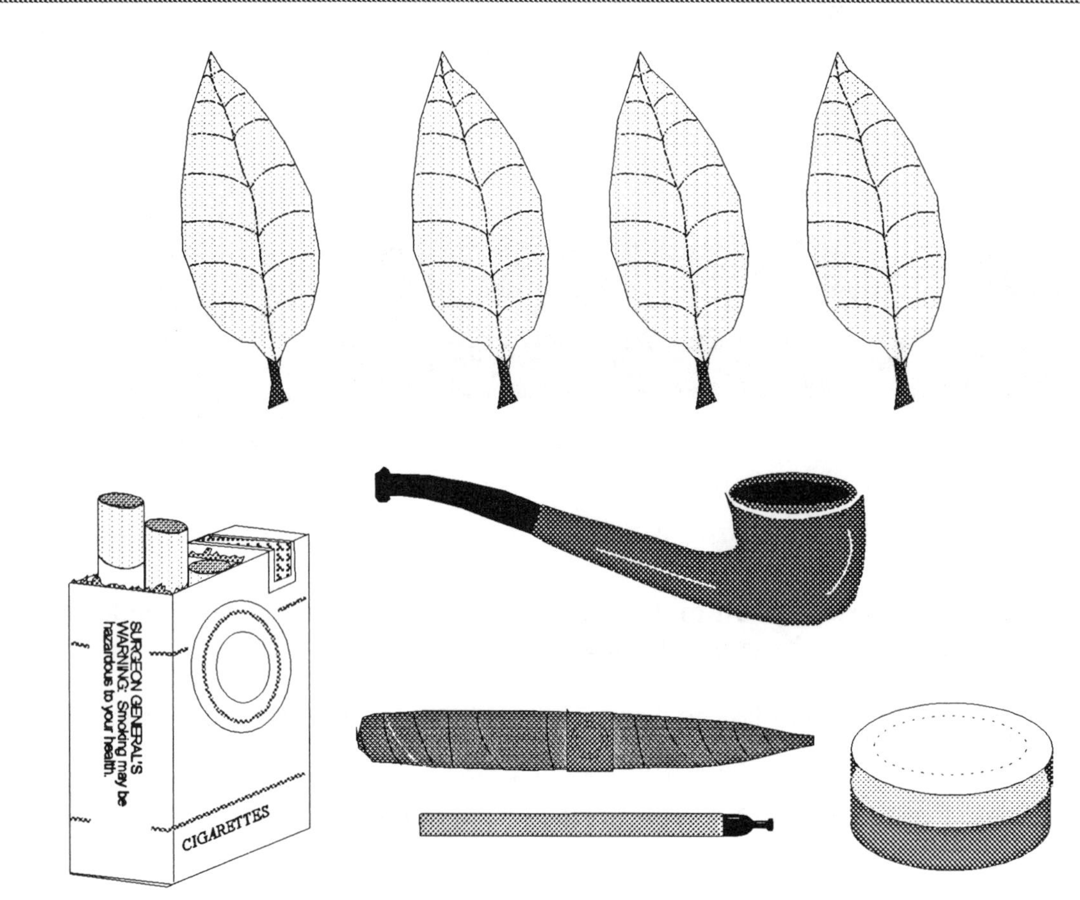

smokeless

TOBACCO

nicotine

carbon monoxide

tars -- carcinogens

12-1

SMOKING -- A MAJOR HEALTH RISK

Cigarette smoking is the largest preventable cause of illness and premature death in America.

The harmful effects of tobacco use were not well known until the early 1960s. The U.S. Surgeon General issued the first major report in 1964.

Tobacco use in **all its forms** is now a significant threat to life.

- Smoking is responsible for more than 450,000 deaths each year. These deaths are all unnecessary.
- 10% of all people will die as a result of smoking-related illnesses.
- The average life expectancy for a chronic smoker is as much as 18 years shorter than for a nonsmoker.
- A 1993 report indicated that each cigarette shortens life by 7 minutes.

12-2

TOBACCO AND HEART DISEASE

NICOTINE
CARBON MONOXIDE
TARS

The risk for heart attack and stroke is 50% to 100% higher for smokers than non-smokers.

Smoking increases:
- heart rate
- blood pressure
- susceptibility to atherosclerosis
- potential for blood clots

Smoking decreases:
- high-density lipoprotein (HDL) cholesterol
- oxygen carrying capacity of the blood

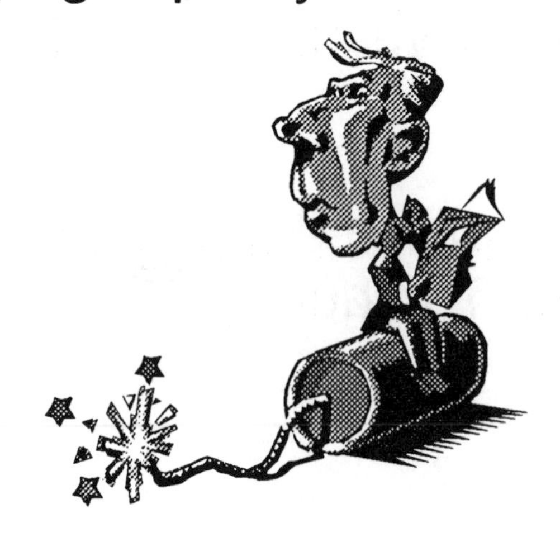

12-3

TOBACCO LAND CANCER

NICOTINE
CARBON MONOXIDE
TARS
carcinogens and co-carcinogens

Tobacco increasesthe risk of cancer:
83% of lung cancer and 30% of all cancers are attributable to smoking.

- lung
- oral cavity
- larynx
- esophagus
- bladder
- pancreas
- kidneys

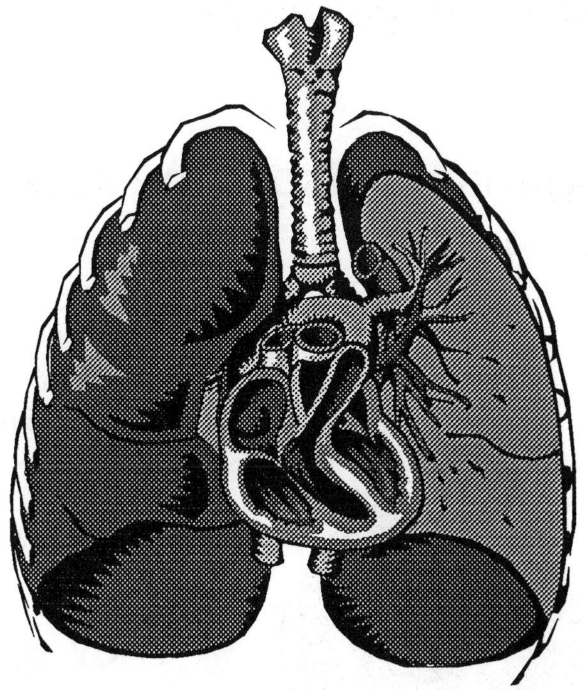

Although half of all cancers are curable, the 5-year survival rate for lung cancer is less than 13%.

Tobacco induced cancers kill about 142,000 people each year.

12-4

OTHER PROBLEMS ASSOCIATED WITH TOBACCO

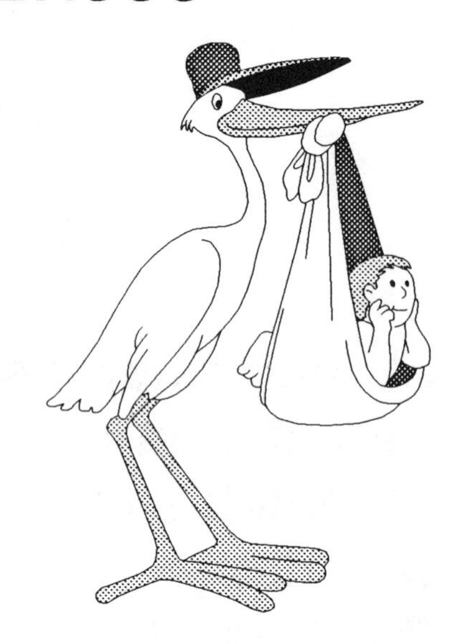

Cigarettesmoking by pregnant women has been linked to:

- retarded fetal growth
- higher risk for spontaneous abortion
- prenatal death

Smoking also is the most prevalentcause of injury and death from fire.

- American business and industry pays more than $16 billion each year as a direct result of smoking in the work-place.
- They also pay another $37 billion in lost productivity because of illness, disability, and death.
- The estimated cost to business for health care each year is between $624 and $4,611 per smoking employee.

12-5
13-1

SMOKING CESSATION

Quitting cigarettes smoking is not easy:

- Only about 20% of smokers who try to quit the first time succeed.

- Even though difficult, it CAN BE DONE!
  More than 95% of successful ex-smokers have quit on their own:
  -- some by quitting cold turkey
  -- some using self-help kits
  -- Others have had professional help

The following seven-step plan has helped many people stop smoking in 4 weeks.

1. Decide positively that you want to quit.
2. Begin a personal diet and exercise program.
3. Decide on the approach you will use.
4. Keep a daily log of your smoking habit.
5. Set the target date for quitting.
6. Stock up on low-calorie foods, drink plenty of water.
7. Do not keep cigarettes handy, stay away from friends who smoke.

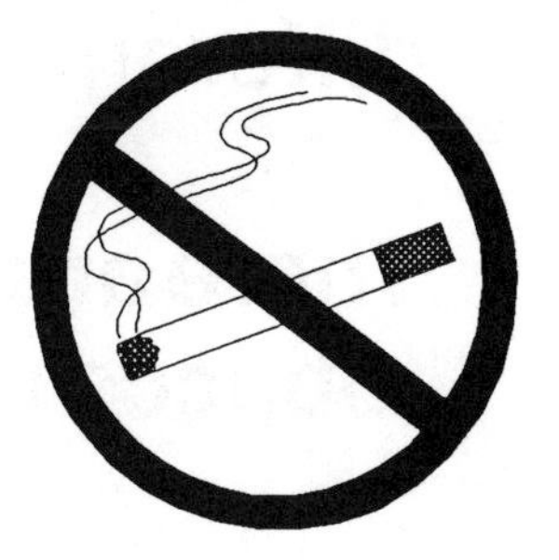

12-6

WHY DO PEOPLE SMOKE?

People start using tobacco for many different reasons, the three most common are:

- peer pressure,
- the desire to appear "grown up,"
- rebellion against authority.

People typically begin to smoke without realizing its detrimental effects.

- Smoking only three packs of cigarettes is enough to cause addiction.
- Smoking is the most widespread example of drug dependency.

People continue to use tobacco for many different reasons.

There are also many different patterens of tobacco use.

Smoking cessation programs must account for thease differences.

12-7

Addictive Behavior and Sexually Transmitted Disease

13

Expanded Chapter Outline

I. CHEMICAL DEPENDENCY & SEXUALLY TRANSMITTED DISEASES

A. **Chemical dependency and sexually transmitted diseases are two of societies most serious problems.**

B. **Addictive behavior and unprotected sex have ruined and ended millionsof lives.**

ADDICTIVE BEHAVIOR

II. ADDICTION

A. **Jacquelyn Small, psychotherapist and author, defines addiction as a problem of imbalance or unease within the body and mind:**
   1. Addiction has many forms including food, television, work, compulsive shopping, even exercise.
   2. The most serious type of addiction is drug dependency.

B. **FOOD. Some people become addicted to food.**
   1. They eat to release stress or boredom.
   2. They eat to reward themselves for every small personal achievement.

C. **T.V. Great numbers of people are addicted to television.**

D. **WORK. Other individualsbecome addicted to their jobs.**
   1. Work may start out enjoyable, but become an unhealthy addiction.
   2. If it totally consumes your life, you may be becoming a workaholic.

E. **EXERCISE. Exercise can enhance a person's life, but for a few individuals,exercise has become an obsessive behavior.**
   1. Compulsive exercisers express guilt when they miss a day's workout.
   2. They continue to exercise even when injured and recovery is needed.
   3. People who exceed the recommended guidelines for fitness are exercising for reasons other than health.

F. **CAFFEINE. Addiction to caffeine can produce undesirable side effects.**
   1. Excess doses of caffeine can produce:
      a. an abnormally rapid heart rate
      b. abnormal heart rhythms
      c. higher blood pressure
      d. birth defects
      e. higher body temperature
      f. increased secretion of gastric acids leading to stomach problems
      g. symptoms of anxiety, depression, nervousness, and dizziness
   2. The caffeine content of different drinks varies with the product:
      a. a cup of coffee, varies from 65 mg to 180 mg.
      b. Colas beverages range in caffeine from 30 to 60 mg.

G. **Other examples of addictive behaviors include:**
   1. GAMBLING
   2. SEX and PORNOGRAPHY

H. **Recognizing that all forms of addiction are unhealthy, this chapter focuses on the three forms of chemical dependency that are the most self-destructive.**
   1. Marijuana
   2. Cocaine
   3. Alcohol
   4. A fourth, tobacco, has been discussed in the previous chapter.

III. MARIJUANA

A. **Marijuana (pot or grass), is the most widely used illegal drug in the U.S.:**
   1. 64% of Americans between ages 18 and 25 have smoked marijuana.
   2. 23% of those 26 and older have smoked marijuana.
   3. 20 million people in the country use marijuana regularly.

B. **Marijuana is prepared from a mixture of crushed leaves etc. from the hemp plant, cannabis sativa:**
   1. In small doses marijuana has a sedative effect.
   2. Larger doses produce physical and psychic changes.

C. **Modern bio-agriculturaltechniques have altered the marijuana plant.**

1. Forms of marijuana used in the 1960s were milder and the harmful effects of the drug were exaggerated.
2. The drug used today, however, is as much as 10 times stronger.
3. Research today shows marijuana to be a dangerous and harmful drug.

D. The major and most active psychoactive ingredient of marijuana is delta-9-tetrahydrocannabinol (THC).

1. In the 1960s THC content in marijuana ranged from .02% to 2%.
2. Today's THC content averages 4% to 6%, some as high as 20%.
3. The THC content in sinsemilla, a high-potency variety from the seedless female cannabis plant, is approximately 8%.

E. THC reaches the brain within 30 seconds after inhaling.

1. The psychic and physical changes reach a peak in about 2 or 3 minutes.
2. THC is metabolized in the liver to waste metabolites.
3. 30% of it remains in the body a week after it was smoked.
4. 30 days or longer are required to eliminate THC completely.
5. The drug always remains in the system of regular users.

F. Some of the short-term effects of marijuana include:

1. Tachycardia (faster heart rate--up to 180 beats per minute.
2. Dryness of the mouth.
3. Reddening of the eyes.
4. Enhanced appetite.
5. Less coordination.
6. Difficulty concentrating.
7. Intermittent confusion.
8. Impairment of short-term memory.
9. Loss of continuity of speech.
10. Interference with the learning process during intoxication.
11. Loss of motivation and interest (amotivational syndrome).

G. Long-term harmful effects include:

1. Atrophy of the brain, leading to irreversible brain damage.
2. Decreased resistance to infectious diseases.
3. Chronic bronchitis.
4. Lung cancer (it contains more hydrocarbons than cigarette smoke).
5. Sterility and impotence.

H. A common myths is that marijuana does not lead to addiction.

1. Ample scientific evidence shows clearly that regular marijuana users do develop physical and psychological dependence.
2. Regular users going without the drug have experiences similar to cigarette smokers.
   a. they crave the substance
   b. go through changes in mood

c. are irritable and nervous
d. become obsessed with getting more "pot"

IV. COCAINE

A. Cocaine was thought for many years to be a relatively harmless drug.

1. Then a new form, crack cocaine, came on the scene.
2. People started dying suddenly following a crack cocaine overdose.
3. Crack cocaine is particularly dangerous and addicting.
4. Cocaine has become the fastest growing drug problem in the U.S.
5. About 5,000 people try cocaine for the first time each day.
6. An estimated 4 to 8 million Americans use cocaine.
7. Most cocaine users have used marijuana previously.

B. Cocaine is a crystalline powder extracted from the leaves of the cocoa plant.

1. (2-beta-carbomethoxy-3-betabenozoxytropane) is the primary psychoactive ingredient.
2. The drug is typically sniffed or snorted, but it can be smoked or injected.
3. Crack is manufactured by mixing it with ammonia. baking soda, and water and heating it until the hydrochlorides evaporate.
4. Users pay more than $2,000 per ounce for cocaine, used in medical therapy it costs about $100 per ounce.
5. Because of the high cost, cocaine is viewed as a luxury drug.

C. Many users are well-educated, affluent, upwardly mobile professionals who otherwise are law-abiding citizens.

1. They begin with a desire to get high at a social gathering.
2. The user will enter an immediate state of euphoria.
3. About one in five will continue to use the drug, some now and then, others for a lifetime of nightmares.

D. When cocaine is snorted, it is absorbed quickly through the mucous membranes of the nose into the bloodstream.

1. The drug usually is arranged in lines one to two inches long.
2. Each line results in about 30 minutes of stimulation.
   a. cocaine seems to help relieve fatigue and increase energy.
   b. it decrease the need for appetite and sleep.
3. Following this stimulation comes a "crash," a state of physiological and psychological depression.
   a. this often leaves the user with the desire to get more.
   b. this can lead to a constant craving for the drug.

E. Addiction becomes a lifetime illness.

1. The individual recovers only by completely abstaining from the drug. A single

pitfall often results in renewed addiction.

2. Sustained cocaine snorting can lead to:
   a. a constant runny nose
   b. nasal congestion and inflammation
   c. perforation of the nasal septum
3. High doses of cocaine can cause:
   a. nervousness
   b. dizziness
   c. blurred vision
   d. vomiting
   e. tremors
   f. seizures
   g. high blood pressure
   h. strokes, angina, and cardiac arrhythmias
4. Long-term consequences of cocaine use include:
   a. loss of appetite and digestive disorders
   b. malnutrition and weight loss
   c. insomnia
   d. confusion, anxiety, paranoia, and hallucinations
5. Freebase (a purer, more potent smokable form of cocaine) users have a higher risk for lung disease.
6. Intravenous users are at risk for hepatitis, AIDS, and other infectious diseases.
7. Large overdoses of cocaine end in sudden death from respiratory paralysis, cardiac arrhythmias, and severe convulsions.

F. Chronic users who crave the drug constantly often turn to crime to sustain their habit.

V. ALCOHOL

A. Alcohol has been used traditionallyfor social occasions and for medical purposes.

1. Alcohol is a staple at parties, ceremonies, dinners, sport contests, etc.
2. It has been used for medical reasons as a mild sedative or pain killer.

B. The psychoactive ingredient in alcoholic beverages is ethyl alcohol.

1. It is a depressant drug that slows down central nervous system activity.
2. It has strong addictive properties and therefore can be abused easily.
3. Alcohol abuse is one of the most significant health-related drug problems.
   a. approximately 1000 million Americans adults (60%) are drinkers.
   b. about 10 million of them will have a drinking problem.
   c. another 3 million teenagers have a drinking problem.

C. The addiction to alcohol develops slowly.

1. Most people who have a drinking problem do not realize it.
2. They become alcoholics when their physical and emotional dependence on the drug, is characterized by constant preoccupation with drinking.

3. Alcohol abuse leads to mental, emotional, physical, and social problems.

D. Many health problems are associated with short-term alcohol consumption.
1. Some problems may be associated each period of intoxication.
2. Other problems are the use of chronic alcohol consumption.
3. Some of the health problems include:
   a. reduced peripheral vision
   b. decreased visual and hearing acuity
   c. slowed reaction time
   d. impaired concentration and motor performance
   e. it dissipates fear
   f. increased risk-taking behaviors
   g. stimulated urination
   h. induced sleep
   i. decreased sexual function
4. An unpleasant and life-threatening effect of drinking is the synergistic action of alcohol when combined with other drugs.
   a. the effects of mixing alcohol with another depressant drug can be much greater than the sum of two drug actions by themselves.
   b. the effects range from loss of consciousness to death.

E. Long-term effects of alcohol abuse may be life-threatening.
1. Some of these detrimental effects are:
   a. cirrhosis of the liver
   b. oral, esophageal, and liver cancer
   c. cardiomyopathy (a disease that affects the heart muscle)
   d. higher blood pressure
   e. greater risk for strokes
   f. inflammation of the pancreas esophagus, stomach, small intestine
   g. stomach ulcers
   h. sexual impotence
   i. malnutrition
   j. loss of memory
   k. psychosis, depression, and hallucinations

VI. ALCOHOL ON CAMPUSES

A. Alcohol is the number-one drug problem among college students:
1. Approximately 86.9% of college students reported using alcohol.
2. 41% of them engage in binge drinking (5 or more drinks).
3. Alcohol is a factor in about 28% of all college dropouts.
4. Today's student spends more on alcohol than on books.
5. Grade-point average (GPA) is related to the number of drinks per week.
6. 36% indicated that they drive while intoxicated.

7. 2% to 3% of college students will die from alcohol-related causes.

B. Excessive drinking can lead to unplanned and unprotected sex (risking HIV infection) or even date rape.

VII. HOW TO CUT DOWN YOUR DRINKING

A. The questionnaire "Alcohol Abuse: Are You Drinking Too Much," given in Figure 13.2. can be used to find out if drinking is a problem in your life.

B. The first and most important step is to want to cut down:
1. If you want to cut down but find you cannot, you had better accept the probability that alcohol is becoming a serious problem for you.
2. If so, you should seek guidance from your physician or from an organization such as Alcoholics Anonymous.

C. The next few suggestions also may help you cut down on alcohol intake:
1. Set reasonable limits for yourself.
2. Learn to say no.
3. Drink slowly.
4. Dilute your drinks.
5. Do not drink on your own.

D. Treatment of drug (including alcohol) addiction seldom is accomplished without professional guidance and support.

SEXUALLY TRANSMITTED DISEASES

I. SEXUALLY TRANSMITTED DISEASES

A. STDs have reached epidemic proportions in the United States:
1. Of the more than 25 known STDs, some are still incurable.
2. About 25% of all Americans will acquire at least one STD in their lifetime.
3. Each year more than 12 million people are newly infected with STDs, including:
   a. 4.6 million cases of chlamydia
   b. 1.8 million of gonorrhea
   c. 1 million of genital warts
   d. half a million of herpes
   e. nearly 100,000 cases of syphilis
   f. more than 46,648 new cases of AIDS

B. If anyone tests positive for any type of STD, they need to tell anyone with whom you have had sex so he or she can be tested, and treated if necessary.

II. CHLAMYDIA

A. Chlamydia is a bacterial infection:

1. It is spread during vaginal, anal, or oral sex.
2. It is also spread from the vagina to a newborn baby during childbirth.

B. Chlamydia is a major factor in male and female infertility:

1. Because it may have no symptoms, three of four people don't realize they have the disease until it is quite serious.
2. According to the CDC, about 20% of all college students have chlamydia.
3. Symptoms, if present, mimic other STDs, so it can be mistreated.
4. Symptoms of serious infection include:
   a. abdominal pain
   b. fever
   c. nausea
   d. vaginal bleeding
   e. arthritis
5. It can be treated successfully with oral antibiotics.
6. However, treatment will not reverse any damage already done.

III. GONORRHEA

A. Gonorrhea, one of the oldest STDs, also is caused by a bacterial infection.

1. Gonorrhea is transmitted through vaginal, anal, and oral sex.
2. Typical symptoms in men include:
   a. a puslike secretion from the penis
   b. painful urination
3. Most infected women don't have any symptoms at first.
4. When the infection is fairly serious, the symptoms might include:
   a. fever
   b. severe abdominal pain
   c. pelvic inflammatory disease

B. Untreated gonorrhea can produce:

1. Infertility, widespread bacterial infection, heart damage, and arthritis.
2. Blindness in children born to infected women.

C. Gonorrhea is treated successfullywith penicillin and other antibiotics.

IV. PELVIC INFLAMMATORY DISEASE

A. PID is caused most frequently by chlamydia and gonorrhea:

1. PID often develops when the STD spreads to the fallopian tubes, uterus, and ovaries.
2. If symptoms are present they might include:
   a. fever, nausea, vomiting, chills, spotting
   b. heavy bleeding during menstrual periods
   c. pain in the lower abdomen during sexual intercourse, between menstrual periods, or urination
3. Because of no symptoms, many women do not know they have PID.
   a. if the women with PID becomes pregnant, it may result in an ectopic or tubal pregnancy
   b. that pregnancy destroys the embryo and can kill the patient

B. PID is treated with antibiotics, bed rest, sexual abstinence and sometimes surgery.

V. GENITAL WARTS

A. Genital warts are caused by a viral infection:

1. The virus is spread through vaginal, anal, and oral sex, or from the vagina to a newborn baby.
2. Warts show up anywhere from 1-2 months to 8 months after exposure.
3. Warts are found on the penis, around the vagina, and around the anus.
4. The warts may be flat or raised.
5. 20% to 30% of sexually active people in the U.S. are infected with genital warts.

B. Health problems associated with genital warts include:

1. Obstruction of the urethra, vagina, and anus.
2. Higher risk for cancers of the cervix, vulva, or penis.
3. Babies born to infected mothers typically develop warts all over their bodies; therefore, Cesarean sections are recommended.

C. Treatment requires completely removing all warts by:

1. Freezing them with liquid nitrogen.
2. Dissolving them with chemicals.
3. Removing them through electrosurgery or laser surgery.
4. The treatment may have to be repeated several times before it is effective.

VI. HERPES

A. Herpes is one of two STDs that have no known cure.

1. It is caused by the herpes simplex types II virus.
2. Sores appear on the genitals and rectum.
3. In conjunction with the sores, victims usually have a mild fever, swollen glands, and headaches.
4. The symptoms usually disappear within a few weeks, then reoccur again and again throughout life.

B. Herpes is highly contagious, particularlyduring an outbreak.

VII. SYPHILIS

A. Syphilisis caused by a bacterial infection and it progresses though several stages.

1. The Primary Stage is marked by a painless sore that appears approximately 3 weeks after infection.
2. The sore appears where the bacteria entered the body.
3. The sore disappears on its own in a few weeks.
4. The Second Stage is marked by the appearance of other sores within 6 months.
5. The symptoms will again disappear by themselves during the Latent Stage.
6. The Latent Stage, during which the victim is not contagious, may last up to 30 years.
7. During the Third Stage of the disease people may develop paralysis, crippling, blindness, heart disease, brain damage, insanity, and even may die.

B. Penicillinand other antibioticsnow are used to treat syphilis.

VIII. HIV and AIDS

A. AIDS is the most frighteningof all STDs because it has no known cure:

1. AIDS stands for acquired immunodeficiency syndrome.
2. It is the end stage of a deadly infection caused by the human immunodeficiency virus HIV.
3. HIV spreads among individuals who choose to engage in risky behavior such as unprotected sex or the sharing of hypodermic needles.

B. When a person becomes infected with HIV, the virus multipliesin the body:

1. At some point the viruses attack and destroy white blood cells.
2. These cells are part of the immune system which fights disease.
3. As the white cells decreases, the immune system gradually fails.
4. Without the immune system, a person becomes susceptible to opportunistic infections.

C. HIV is a progressive disease:

1. At first, people who become infected with HIV may not know they are infected.
2. An incubation period of weeks, months, or years may go by during which time no

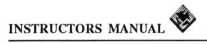

symptoms appear.
3. During this period a person may be HIV positive, but does not yet have AIDS.
4. When the infection progresses to the point at which certain diseases develop, the person is said to have AIDS.
5. HIV itself doesn't kill, nor do people die of AIDS.
6. Death occurs when a weakened immune system is unable to fight off opportunistic diseases.
7. AIDS is the term used to define the final stage of HIV infection.
8. Most of the opportunistic diseases that AIDS patients develop are harmless and rare in the general population but are fatal to the AIDS victim.
9. The two most common fatal conditions in AIDS patients are:
   a. pneumocystis carinii pneumonia (a parasitic infection of the lungs)
   b. kaposis sarcoma (a type of skin cancer)

D. Several years, 7 to 8 on the average, may elapse after infection before the individual develops the symptoms that fit the case definition of AIDS.
1. From that point on, the person may live another 2 to 3 years.
2. Earliest symptoms of the disease include:
   a. unexplained weight loss
   b. constant fatigue
   c. mild fever
   d. swollen lymph glands
   e. diarrhea
   f. sore throat
3. Advanced symptoms include:
   a. loss of appetite
   b. skin diseases
   c. night sweats
   d. deterioration of the mucous membranes causing brain and spinal cord damage

E. An HIV antibody test is the only means to determine whether someone has HIV:
1. Being HIV-positive does not necessarily mean the person has AIDS.
2. On the average, the body requires 3 months to manufacture enough antibodies to show positive in an HIV antibody test.
3. If HIV infection is suspected, a prudent waiting period of 3 to 6 months should be observed before testing.
4. During this waiting period, and from there on, these individuals should refrain from endangering themselves and others further through risky behaviors.

F. HIV is transmitted by the exchange of cellular body fluids:
1. Blood.
2. Semen.
3. Vaginal secretions.
4. Maternal milk.

G. These fluids may be exchanged:

1. During sexual intercourse.
2. By using hypodermic needles used previously by infected individuals.
3. Between an infected woman who is pregnant and her developing fetus.
4. Between an infected mother and her baby during childbirth or during breast feeding.
5. From a blood transfusion or organ transplant. (The risk of being infected with HIV from a blood transfusion today is slight.)

IX. RISKY BEHAVIORS

A. Every time you engage in risky behavior, you run the risk of contracting HIV.

B. The two most basic risky behaviors are:

1. Having unprotected sex with an HIV-infected person.
   a. that includes vaginal, anal, or oral sex.
   b. unprotected sex means having sex without using a condom properly.
   c. only latex condoms that says "disease prevention" on the package should be used.
   d. unprotected anal sex is the riskiest type of sex.
   e. although in most cases bleeding is not visible, anal sex almost always causes tiny tears and bleeding in the rectum.
2. Sharing hypodermic needles with someone who is infected:
   a. following an injection, a small amount of blood remains in the needle and sometimes in the syringe itself.
   b. if the person who used the syringe is infected and someone else uses that same syringe, the virus may be spread.
   c. all used syringes should be destroyed and disposed of immediately after their use.
   d. caution must be taken when getting acupuncture, a tattoo, or the ears pierced.

C. HIV is not transmitted through casual contact. HIV cannot be caught:

1. By spending time with, shaking hands, or hugging an infected person.
2. From a toilet seat, dishes, or silverware used by an HIV patient.
3. By sharing a drink, food, a towel or clothes with an infected person.

X. HIV RISK REDUCTION

A. The following precautions can reduce your risk for getting HIV and AIDS:

1. Postpone sex until you and your uninfected partner are prepared to enter in a lifetime monogamous relationship.
2. Unless you are in a monogamous relationship and you know your partner is not infected, practice safe sex every single time you have sex.

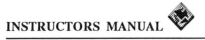

8. Don't share toothbrushes, razors, or other implements that could become contaminated with blood, with anyone who might be infected.
3. Be cautious regarding procedures such as acupuncture, tattooing, and ear piercing, in which needles or other nonsterile instruments may be used.
4. If you are planning to undergo artificial insemination, insist on frozen sperm obtained from a laboratory that tests all donors for infection.
5. If you know you will be having surgery in the near future, and if you are able, consider donating blood for your own use.

B. **Avoidance of risky behaviors that destroy quality of life and life itself are critical components of a healthy lifestyle.**

C. **Learning the facts so you can make responsible choices can protect you and those around you from startlingand unexpected conditions.**

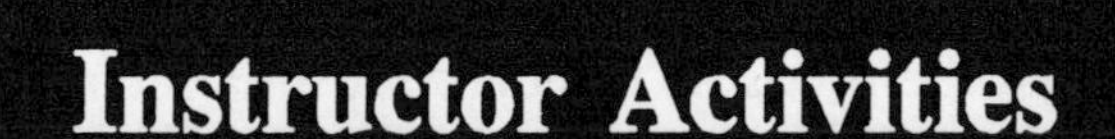

Instructor Activities

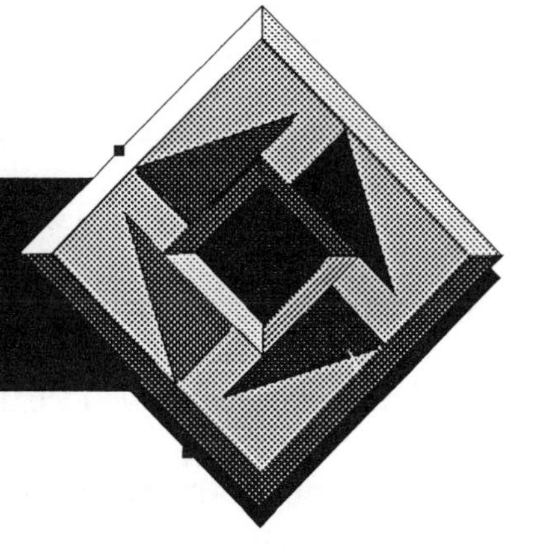

1. **Show overhead transparency** 13-1 revealing only the word addiction at the top. Ask the students to explain what the word means to them. Then reveal the rest of transparency and draw any significance between what the students said and the origin of the word in Roman law.

2. **Show overhead transparency** 13-2 and discuss examples of addiction other than to drugs. Explain that some behaviors that are socially acceptable and even admired can become addictions when taken to the extreme. Point out that in discussing addictions it is risky to over generalize. Although some types of addiction are far worse than others, they all have some common characteristics.

3. **Show overhead transparency** 13-3 and discuss the addiction problems associated with marijuana. Refer to Section III of the expanded outline.

4. **Show overhead transparency** 13-4 and discuss the addiction problems associated with cocaine. Refer to Section IV of the expanded outline.

5. **Show overhead transparency** 13-5 and discuss the addiction problems associated with alcohol. Refer to Section V of the expanded outline.

6. **Show overhead transparency** 13-6 and discuss the things that people can do to help themselves or help someone else with an addiction problem. Emphasize the need for professional help.

7. **Write on the chalkboard** the following words: virus, bacteria, yeast, arthropod. Point out that sexually transmitted diseases are caused by viruses and bacteria that are so fragile that they can't exist outside of the protective environment of the human body. People should not be to frightened by STDs because they are spread primarily through one process, intimate sexual contact. We know how they are spread and we know how to protect ourselves against them. If we follow the steps to protect ourselvs from the STDs, we have a greater reason to fear other disease-producing organisms which are more hardy and more prevalent in our environment.

   Before the polio vaccine, people were very frightened by the polio epidemics that left many people dead and crippled. They did not know how they contacted the polio virus for it could be almost anywhere. They did not know how to prevent it for it was not associated with any particular behavior. At first there was no standardized treatment. But with STDs, particularly AIDS, we know the consequence and we know how to prevent it, yet millions of people are unwilling to accept those preventive measures. Ask the students, why do you think this is?

8. **Show overhead transparency** 13-7 through 13-12 from this instructor's manual and discuss the pertinent characteristics of the various STDs discussed in this text.

   Chlamydia, Gonorrhea, Syphilis, Herpes, HIV-AIDS, and others.

9. **Discuss** points presented in Sections IX and X on Risk Behaviors and Risk Reduction.

ADDICTION

WORD ORIGIN:

Rome

Addictus — A debtor awarded as a slave to his or her creditors.

Addicere — To bind a person over to one thing or another.

Today

Addict — One who is a slave to a behavior or substance.

Some estimates are that well over 30% of all Americans are addicts of some kind.

13-1

EXAMPLES OF ADDICTION

Drugs
To escape or alter perception.

Gambling
For the excitement of taking a risk.

Risk Taking
The thrill of putting life in danger.

Violence
The thrill of hurting other people.

Sex
Sensual stimulation and escape.

Eating
A substitute for affection.
Sensual gratification.

Sleeping
To escape life's problems.

Shopping
A reaction to disappointment.

Exercising
To produce endorphins and euphoria.

Working
For acclaim or to avoid other responsibilities.

Watching TV
To escape.
To maintain sensory stimulation.

Traits
Compulsive nervous traits.

13-2

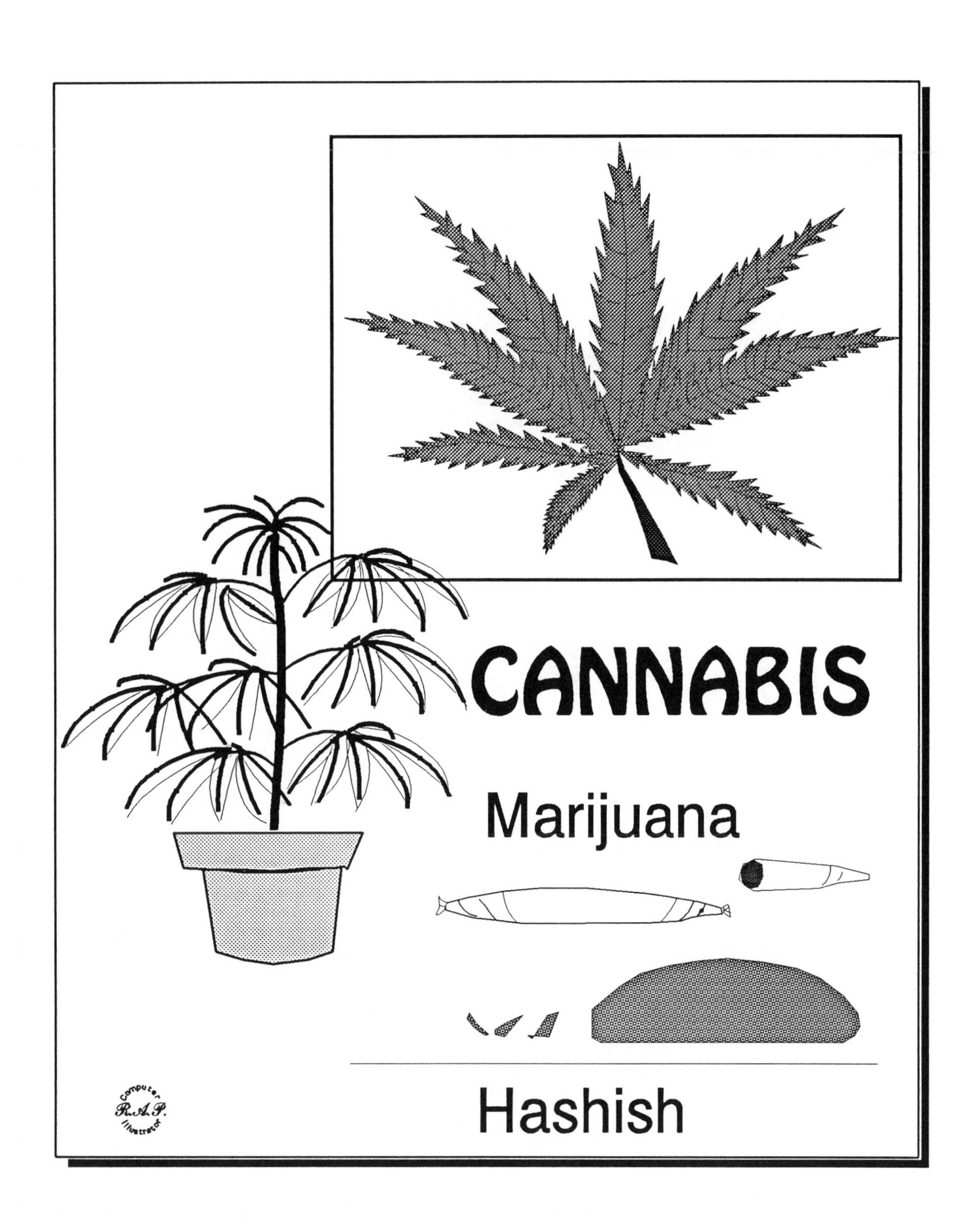

13-3

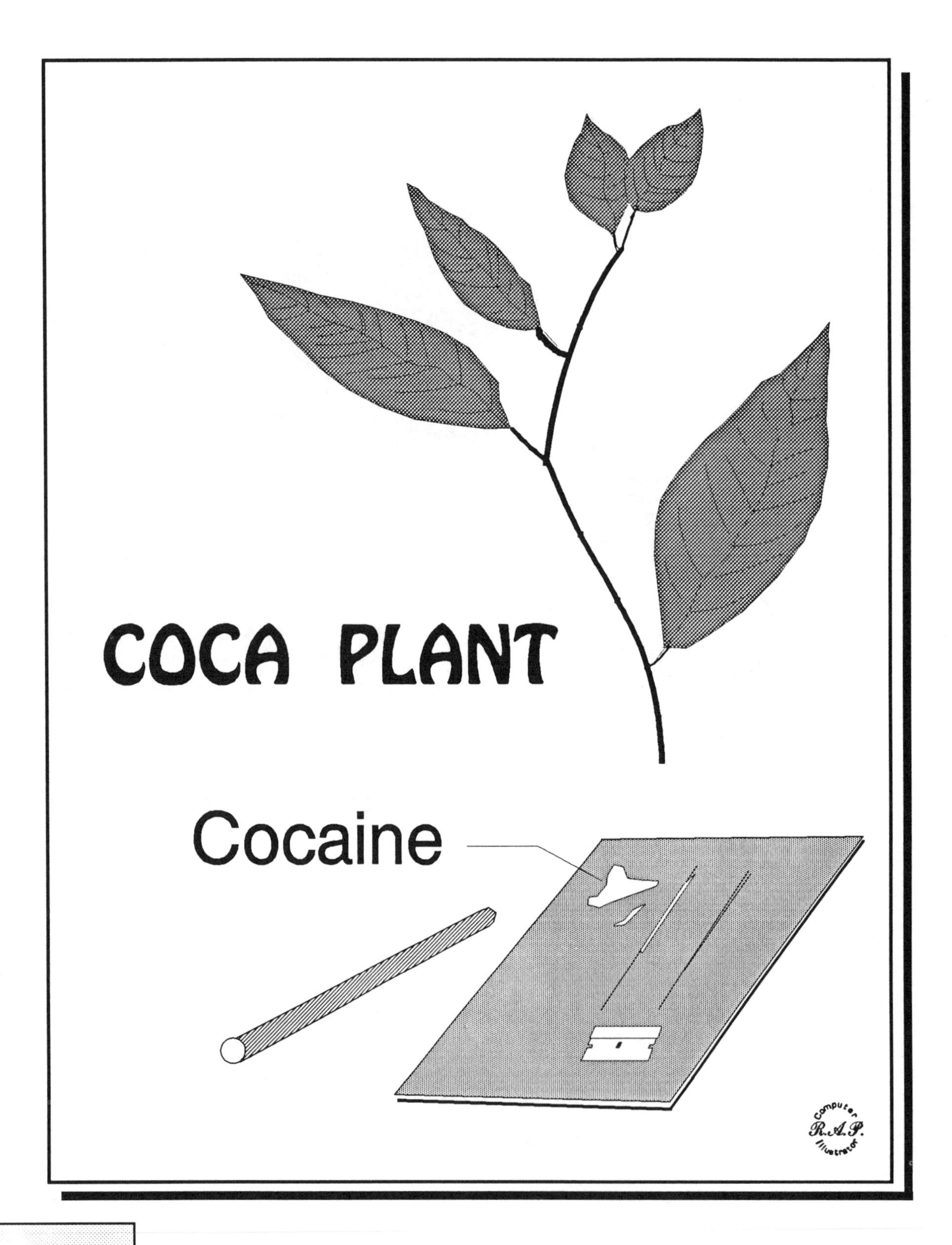

13-4

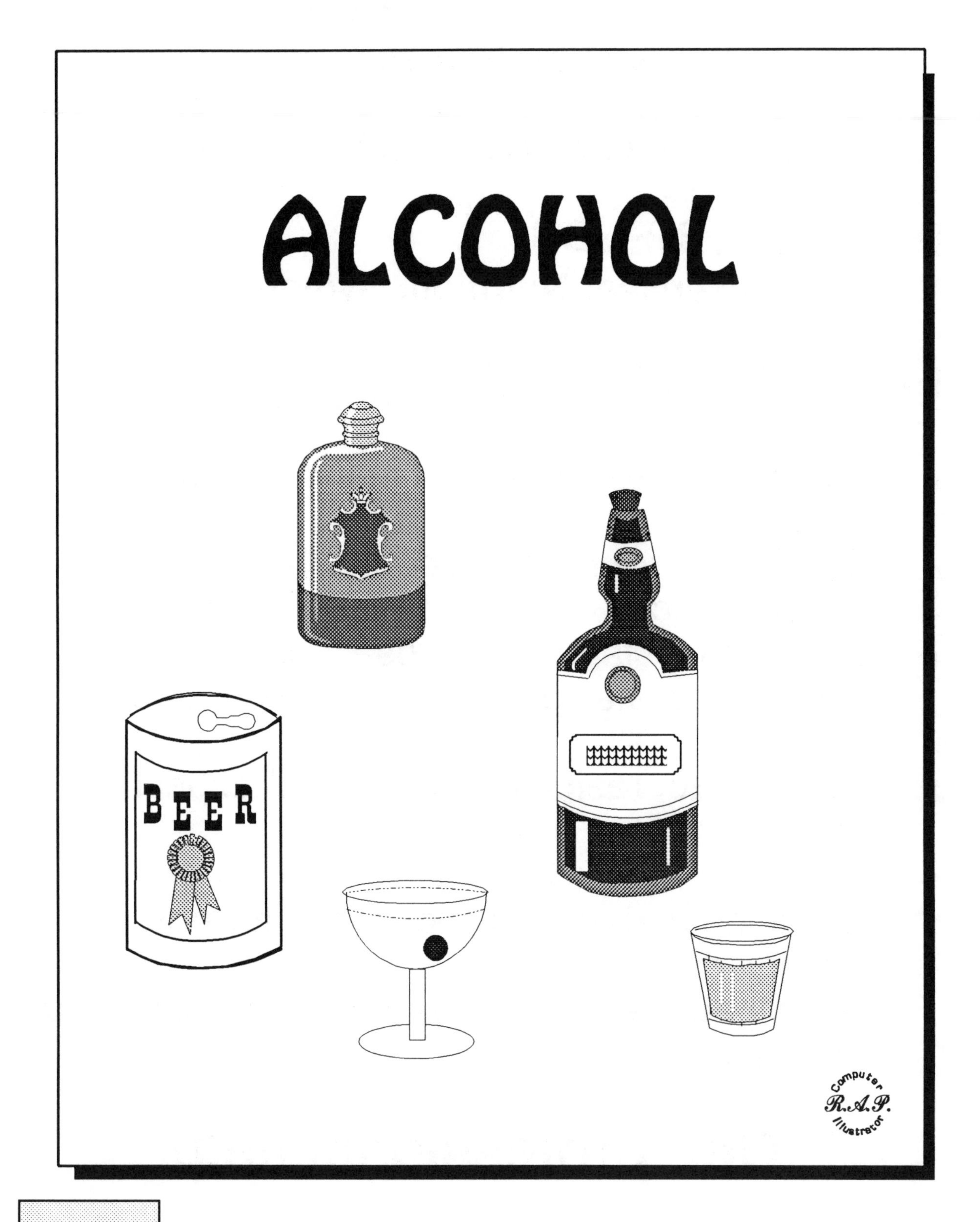

13-5

HOW TO HELP

Yourself or Someone Else

Find better ways to meet basic needs

PHYSICAL NEEDS

Rest, Exercise, Nutrition, Hygiene

EMOTIONAL NEEDS

- **Self-esteem**—get involved in things that bring success.
- **Confront Problem**—recognize the consequences of the behavior.
- **Avoid associated patterns**—Select alternatives, stay away from the associated patterns.
- **Commit to realistic goals**—don't expect too much at once.
- **Visualize Rewards**—see the benefits of changing and the consequences for not changing.
- **Anticipate Relapses**—learn from mistakes and keep trying.

Get professional help

13-6

CHLAMYDIA

4,000,000

CAUSE	*chlamydia trachomatous bacterium* (acts like a virus)
INCUBATION	1 to 2 weeks
SYMPTOMS	Like gonorrhea: Painful urination, penial or vaginal discharge, abdominal pain, genital itches. ♂ 10% asymptomatic ♀ 60% - 10% asymptomatic
COMPLICATIONS	♀ Leading cause of PID, ectopic pregnancy, infertility, miscarriages, sterility (10%).
	♂ Prostatitis, urinary tract infection.
	Infants: eye infection, blindness, pneumonia.
DIAGNOSIS	Culture of cervical smear
COMMUNICABLE	Throughout infection until treatment.
TREATMENT	Antibiotics, (reliable if caught early)

13-7

GONORRHEA

1,500,000

CAUSE	*neisseria gonorrhea bacterium*
INCUBATION	2 to 7 days
SYMPTOMS	♂ Painful and difficult urination, penial discharge.
	♀ **Early**: 60% asymptomatic. **Late**: Painful urination, vaginal discharge, abnormal menses.
	Sore throat -- oral sex Rectal pain -- anal sex
COMPLICATIONS	♀ PID (pelvic inflammatory disease), ectopic pregnancy, sterility. ♂ sterility **Infants**: eye infection, blindness.
DIAGNOSIS	Smear and lab culture. Treatment is often based on history without diagnosis.
COMMUNICABLE	Throughout infection until treatment.
TREATMENT	Antibiotics, (reliable for standard strains) *cefixime* for new strains

13-8

SYPHILIS

120,000

CAUSE		*treponema palladium* spirochete bacteria
INCUBATION		3 to 6 weeks
SYMPTOMS	2 weeks	**PRIMARY:** Chancre sore at point of contact -- genital, oral, anal Symptoms disappear.
	6 weeks	**none**
	10 weeks	**SECONDARY:** Fever, rash, lesions, hair loss. Symptoms disappear, may reappear
	10 yrs	**LATENT: none**
	20 yrs	**TERTIARY:** Inflammation and damage to any body tissue. (see complications)
COMPLICATIONS		Blindness, deafness, crippling, paralysis, aneurysms, brain damage (paresis), death. **CONGENITAL:** death and deformity
DIAGNOSIS		Smear, blood test, spinal tap. (false positive possible)
COMMUNICABLE		2 to 3 years (congenital longer).
TREATMENT		Penicillin, (very large dose) (reliable in early stages)

13-9

HERPES SIMPLEX—2

500,000

CAUSE	*herpes simplex virus type II*
INCUBATION	10 days
SYMPTOMS	Slight fever, tingling, pain, swollen lymph glands, painful blisters on genital and anal area. Symptoms subsides and recur periodically. Asymptomatic while dormant.
COMPLICATIONS	Linked to cervical cancer. **Infants:** CNS damage, death.
DIAGNOSIS	Blisters, cultures,
COMMUNICABLE	By body secretions, close contact (not necessarily intercourse). **Infants:** during delivery (Caesarean delivery may be advised)
TREATMENT	**No Cure.** *Acycovir* tablets for symptom relief.

13-10

HIV—AIDS

50,000

CAUSE	*HIV virus*
INCUBATION	HIV 3 to 6 months AIDS 7 to 10 years later
SYMPTOMS	**EARLY:** Fatigue, weight loss, low-grade fever, swollen lymph glands, sore throat diarrhea. **LATE:** Loss of appetite, night sweats, deterioration of skin and membranes.
COMPLICATIONS	Crippled immune system. Autoimmune diseases. Susceptible to many diseases. Death from opportunistic diseases.
DIAGNOSIS	HI blood test. Positive for antibodies.
COMMUNICABLE	Body secretions: semen, blood, needles. Genital, anal, oral sex,
TREATMENT	**No Cure.** For symptoms.

13-11

OTHER STDs

Genital Warts

Viral Hepatitis Type B

Pelvic Inflammatory Disease

Pubic Lice

Scabies

Chancroid

Lymphogranuloma

Granuloma Inguinal

Yeast Infections

Trichomoniasis

Human Papilloma Virus

Non-Gonoccal Urethritis

Etc. (to total about 25)

13-12

Healthy Lifestyle Issues and Wellness Guideliens for the Future

14

Expanded Chapter Outline

I. GUIDELINES FOR FUTURE

A. This lesson focuses on three factors involved in daily living that have not already been discussed:

1. Spirituality.
2. Exercise and aging.
3. Health-promoting behaviors.

B. Guidelines for consumer choices are also focuses of this lesson:

1. This includes selecting a health/fitness club.
2. It also deals with organizing an exercise programs within your home.

C. This lesson will also give some practical guidelines for:

1. Determining how well you are achieving your wellness objectives.
2. Charting a personal wellness program for the future.

II. SPIRITUAL WELL-BEING

A. One definition of spiritualwell-being that encompasses Christiansand non-Christians alike, indicates that spiritualwell-being as an affirmation of life in a relationshipwith God, self, community, and environment that nurtures and celebrates wholeness.

1. This definition assumes that all people are spiritual in nature.
2. Spiritual health provides a unifying power that integrates the other dimensions of wellness.
3. Basic characteristics of spiritual people include:
   a. a sense of meaning and direction in life
   b. a relationship to a higher being
   c. closeness to others
   d. freedom

e. prayer, faith, and love
f. peace, fulfillment and joy
g. altruism (service to others)

4. Spiritual influences associated with religion have been a major part of cultures since the beginning of time:
   a. One recent survey found that 94% of the U.S. population believes in some form of God or universal spirit.
   b. Many people believe that a relationship with God can be meaningful.
   c. God can grant help, guidance, and assistance in daily living.
   d. Our mortal existence has a purpose.

B. If we accept any or all of these statements, spiritual attainments will have a definite effect on our happiness and well-being.

III. SPIRITUALITY AND HEALTH

A. The relationship between spirituality and health is more difficult to establish scientifically than other lifestyle factors.

1. Several research studies have reported positive relationships among spiritual well-being, emotional well-being, and life's satisfaction.
2. People who attend church and participate in religious organizations:
   a. regularly enjoy better health
   b. have a lower incidence of chronic diseases
   c. handle stress more effectively
   d. seem to live longer
3. Although the reasons why religious affiliation enhances wellness are difficult to determine, possible reasons include:
   a. the promotion of healthy lifestyle behaviors
   b. social support
   c. assistance in times of crisis
   d. counseling to overcome one's weaknesses
4. Researchers have found that most successful men and women:
   a. have strong spiritual values
   b. have experienced a crisis early in life
   c. seemed to be helped in the crisis by their spiritual beliefs

B. Altruism, a key attribute of spiritual people, seems to enhance health and longevity.

1. Altruism is defined as true concern for the welfare of others or a sincere desire to serve others above one's personal needs.
2. Researchers believe that doing good for others is good for oneself.
3. Helping others is especially good for the immune system.

C. Wellness requires a balance between physical, mental, spiritual, emotional, and social well-being.

1. The relationship between spirituality and wellness, therefore, is meaningful in our

quest for a better quality of life.

2. Optimum spirituality requires development of the spiritual nature to its fullest potential.

IV. EXERCISE AND AGING

A. The elderly population is the fastest growing segment of the American society.

1. In 1880, less than 3% of the total population was older than 65.
2. By 1980 the elderly population had reached 11.3% of the population.
3. By 2035, the elderly will make up 20% of the total population.

B. Fitness is just as important for older people as it is for young people.

1. Older individuals who are physically fit also enjoy better health and a higher quality of life.
2. The main objective of fitness programs for older adults should be to help them improve their functional health status.
3. This implies the ability to maintain independent living status and avoiding disability.

C. Relationship Between Fitness and Aging:

1. There is generally a decline in physical capacity as people age.
   a. there is no hard evidence to prove that the decline is related primarily to the aging process.
   b. reduced physical capacity may be more closely associated with the lack of physical activity than with the effects of aging.
   c. data on individuals who maintained a systematic physical activity program throughout life indicate that they did not experience the typical decline in later years.
2. Unhealthy behaviors precipitate premature aging:
   a. from a functional point of view, the typical sedentary American is about 25 years older than his or her chronological age.
   b. an active 60-year-old person can have a work capacity similar to that of a sedentary 40-year-old.
   c. for sedentary people, productive life ends at about age 60.
   d. these people stop living at age 60, but are not buried until several years later.
3. Scientists believe a healthy lifestyle allows people to live a vibrant, independent life until approximately age 95.
   a. then when death comes, it usually is rather quick and not as a result of prolonged illness.
   b. such are the rewards of a wellness way of life.

D. Physical Training in the Older Adult:

1. Older adults who increase their level of physical activity experience significant changes in:
   a. cardiovascular endurance

b. strength
c. flexibility

2. The extent of the changes depends on their initial fitness level and the types of activities selected (walking, cycling, strength training).
   a. improvements in older adults are similar to those of younger people, although older people require a longer training period to achieve these changes.
   b. declines in endurance per decade of life after age 25 is about 9% for sedentary adults and 5% or less in active people.
3. Older adults can increase their strength, but the amount of muscle hypertrophy decreases with age.
   a. strength gains close to 200% have been found in previously inactive adults over age 90.
   b. isometric and other intense weight-training exercises should be avoided.
   c. older adults should participate in activities that require continuous and rhythmic muscular activity at about 50% to 70% of functional capacity.

V. AN EDUCATED WELLNESS CONSUMER

A. Quackery has infiltrated the fitness and wellness programs.

1. The rapid growth of the fitness and wellness movement during the last two decades has spurred the promotion of fraudulent fitness products.
2. Many consumers are deceived by promises of *miraculous, quick, and easy* ways toward total well-being.
3. Today's market is saturated with *special* foods, diets, supplements, equipment, books, and videos that promise quick, dramatic results.

B. Quackery and fraud have been defined as the conscious promotion of unproven claims for profit.

1. Advertisements are often are based on:
   a. testimonials
   b. unproven claims
   c. secret research
   d. half-truths
2. The advertisements are filled with quick-fix statements that the uneducated consumer wants to hear.
   a. large and small enterprise make a large profit from the consumers' willingness to pay for spectacular solutions to problems they have brought on by their unhealthy lifestyle.
   b. television, magazine, and newspaper advertisements, programs, and articles are not necessarily reliable.

C. Three problems became apparent to the educated consumer.

1. First, there is no such thing as spot-reducing; therefore, the claims could not be true.

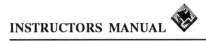

2. Second, 5 minutes of daily exercise burn hardly any calories and, therefore, have no effect on weight loss.
3. Third, the intended abdominal (gut) muscles were not really involved during the exercise.

D. Even though deceit is all around us, we can protect ourselves from consumer fraud.

1. The first step, of course, is education.
   a. you have to be an informed consumer of the product you intend to purchase.
   b. if you do not have or cannot find the answers, seek the advice of a reputable professional.
   c. ask someone who understands the product but does not stand to profit from the transaction.
   d. also, be alert to those who bill themselves as "experts." Look for qualifications and credentials.
2. Another clue to possible fraud is, if it sounds too good to be true, it probably is.
   a. when claims are made, ask where the claims are published.
   b. newspapers, magazines, and trade books are apt to be unreliable sources of information.
   c. refereed scientific journals are the most reliable sources of information.

E. To avoid misinformationand fraud, you should try to stay up to date on fitness and wellness developments.

1. You should buy a reputable and updated fitness/wellness book every 4 to 5 years.
2. To stay current you might also subscribe to a credible health, fitness, nutrition, or wellness newsletter.

VI. HEALTH/FITNESS CLUB MEMBERSHIPS

A. If you have mastered the contents of this book, you should be able to maintain an excellent fitness program within your home and neighborhood. You need not join a health club.

B. However, for a variety of reasons you may want to consider joining a health/fitness facility. If so:

1. Examine all exercise options in your community: health clubs, YMCAs, gyms, colleges, schools, community centers, senior centers, etc.
2. Check to see if the facility's atmosphere is pleasurable and non-threatening to you.
3. Find out what types of facilities are available: track, courts, aerobic exercise room, strength training room, treadmills, bicycle ergometers, pool, saunas, hot tubs, locker rooms, etc. Make sure the facilities and equipment meet your activity interests..
4. Analyze costs versus facilities, equipment, and programs. Take a look at your personal budget. Will you really use the facility?
5. Consider the location. Is the facility close, or do you have to travel several miles to get there? Distance often discourages participation.

6. Check on times the facility is accessible. Is it open during your preferred exercise time?
7. Work out at the facility several times before becoming a member. Are people standing in line to use the equipment?
8. Inquire about the instructors' qualifications. Do the fitness instructors have college degrees or professional certifications? Do the instructors spend time with members?
9. Consider the approach to fitness. Is it well-rounded?
10. Ask about supplementary services. Does the facility provide for regular health and fitness assessments? Are wellness seminars (nutrition, weight control, stress management) offered? Do these have hidden costs?

C. You may consider purchasing your own exercise equipment.

1. Many people buy expensive equipment only to find out they really do not enjoy that mode of activity.
2. Recognize the limitations of the equipment.
3. Actually try out the piece of equipment several times first.
4. Also consider the quality of the equipment. Some cheaper brands of equipment may not be durable, so your investment would be wasted.

VII. SELF-EVALUATION AND BEHAVIORAL OBJECTIVES FOR THE FUTURE

A. The main objective of this course is to provide the information and experiences necessary to implement your personal fitness and wellness program.

B. You have learned that self-evaluation is important and you have had an opportunity to assess various fitness and wellness components and write behavioral objectives to improve your quality of life.

C. You now should take the time to evaluate how well you have achieved your own objectives.

D. The real challenge will come now that you are about to finish this course. Adhering to a program in a structured setting is a lot easier than it will be from now on when you will be on your own.

VIII. A CHALLENGE FOR THE FUTURE

A. The process of change is never easy. Lifestyle behaviors are developed over many years.

B. The real challenge will come now: a lifetime commitment to fitness and wellness. To make the commitment easier, enjoy yourself and have fun along the way.

Instructor Activities

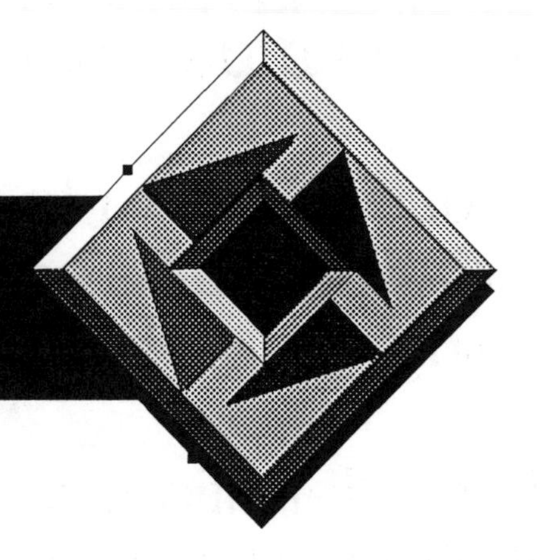

1. **Use overhead transparency** 14-1 and 14-2 to discuss the influence of spiritual well-being on health and wellness.

2. **Use overhead transparency** 14-3 to discuss benefits of lifelong fitness and wellness programs as related to aging.

3. **Use overhead transparency** 14-4 to discuss the problems of quackery, fraud, and misinformation within the wellness and fitness movement.

4. **Show overhead transparency** 14-1 as a concluding course comment.

SPIRITUAL WELL-BEING

The philosophical base of most world religious provide a definition spiritual well-being.

Those who turn to other sources, such as nature, for affirmation also find a sense of spiritual well-being.

Such definitions include the following ideas:

- Spiritual well-being is an confirmation of the values that define our relationship with God, self, community, and environment.

- Spiritual well-being nurtures and celebrates our wholeness and provides a unifying power that integrates the other dimensions of wellness.

- All people are spiritual by nature.

Basic characteristics of spiritual people include:

- a sense of meaning and direction in life
- a relationship to a higher power or influence
- closeness and service to others (altruism)
- freedom, faith, prayer, love, peace, fulfillment, joy

14-1

SPIRITUAL INFLUENCES

Spiritual influences associated with religion have been a major part of cultures since the beginning of time. One recent survey found that 94% of the U.S. population believes they have a relationship with some form of God or universal spirit. Many people believe that such a relationship can:

- It gives our life direction and purpose.
- Provide guidance and assistance in daily living.

Several research studies have reported positive relationships between physical health and spiritual well-being. People who participate regularly in religious activities:

- handle stress more effectively
- enjoy better health and live longer
- have a lower incidence of chronic diseases

This is particularly true in those religious organizations which:

- promote healthy lifestyle behaviors
- provide social support
- provide assistance in times of crisis
- provide confidential counseling
- provide opportunities for altruistic service

14-2

EXERCISE AND AGING

Fitness is just as important for older people as it is for young people.

Older individuals who are physically fit also enjoy better health and a higher quality of life.

The main objective of fitness programs for older adults should be to help them:

- Maintain or improve their functional health.
- Avoiding disability.
- Maintain and independent living status.

There is no hard evidence to prove that the general decline in physical capacity as people age is related primarily to the aging process. Reduced physical capacity may be more closely associated with the lack of physical activity.

Data on individuals who maintained a systematic physical activity program throughout life indicate that they did not experience the typical decline in later years.

- An active 60-year-old person can have a work capacity similar to that of a sedentary 40-year-old.
- Scientists believe a healthy lifestyle allows people to live a vibrant, independent life until near age 95.

14-3

QUACKERY
IN THE FITNESS AND WELLNESS MOVEMENT.

Quackery is the conscious promotion of unproven health claims for profit.

Advertisements are filled with misinformation.

The consumer wants a quick-fix.

The rapid growth of the fitness and wellness movement during the last two decades has spurred the promotion of fraudulent fitness products.

- miraculous, quick, and easy ways to fitness
- special foods, diets, and supplements,
- newly engineered physical fitness equipment
- books, and videos that promise dramatic results.

Advertisements are often are based on:

- testimonials
- unproven claims
- secret research
- half-truths

Education is the first step in protecting ourselves from quackery, fraud, and consumer misinformation.

14-4

THE FUTURE

Change is certain, but it need not be frightening.

Be Fit
Be Prepared

The process of change is never easy.

Lifestyle behaviors are developed over many years.

The right lifestyle changes now, will pay bigger and better dividends the longer we live.

Make a lifetime commitment to fitness and wellness.

To make the commitment easier, enjoy yourself and have fun along the way.

14-5